TABLE OF CONTENTS

ABOUT THE AUTHORS

Timothy F. Meiller, DDS, PhD

Dr Meiller is Professor of Oncology and Diagnostic Sciences at the Baltimore College of Dental Surgery and Professor of Oncology in the Program of Oncology at the Greenebaum Cancer Center, University of Maryland Baltimore. He has held his position in Diagnostic Sciences at the Dental School for 34 years and serves as an attending faculty at the Greenebaum Cancer Center.

Dr Meiller is a Diplomate of the American Board of Oral Medicine and a graduate of Johns Hopkins University and the University of Maryland Dental and Graduate Schools, holding a DDS and a PhD in Immunology/Virology. He has over 200 publications to his credit, maintains an active general dental practice, and is a consultant to the National Institutes of Health. He is currently engaged in ongoing investigations into cellular immune dysfunction in oral diseases associated with AIDS, in cancer patients, and in other medically-compromised patients.

Richard L. Wynn, BSPharm, PhD

Richard L. Wynn, PhD, is Professor of Pharmacology at the Baltimore College of Dental Surgery, Dental School, University of Maryland Baltimore. Dr Wynn has served as a dental educator, researcher, and teacher of dental pharmacology and dental hygiene pharmacology for his entire professional career. He holds a BS (pharmacy; registered pharmacist, Maryland), an MS (physiology) and a PhD (pharmacology) from the University of Maryland. Dr Wynn chaired the Department of Pharmacology at the University of Maryland Dental School from 1980 to 1995. Previously, he chaired the Department of Oral Biology at the University of Kentucky College of Dentistry.

Dr Wynn has to his credit over 300 publications including original research articles, textbooks, textbook chapters, monographs, and articles in continuing education journals. He has given over 500 continuing education seminars to dental professionals in the U.S., Canada, and Europe. Dr Wynn has been a consultant to the drug industry for 25 years and his research laboratories have contributed to the development of new analgesics and anesthetics. He is a consultant to the Academy of General Dentistry, the American Dental Association, and a former consultant to the Council on Dental Education, Commission on Accreditation. He is a featured columnist and his drug review articles, entitled Pharmacology Today, appear in each issue of General Dentistry, a journal published by the Academy. One of his primary interests continues to be keeping dental professionals informed on all aspects of drug use in dental practice.

Ann Marie McMullin, MD

Dr McMullin is board certified in emergency medicine and departed the Cleveland Clinic Foundation Emergency Department after 7 years to take a position with the U.S. Navy as civilian staff in the emergency department, U.S. Naval Hospital, Rota, Spain. She is a graduate of the University of Illinois, Champaign/Urbana, and obtained her medical degree from the University of Illinois College of Medicine, Peoria. Dr McMullin completed a transitional internship at Saint Mary's Medical Service in Grand Rapids, Michigan, and subsequently spent three years as a General Medical Officer in the United States Navy. For two of these years, Dr McMullin worked in the Emergency Department at the Naval Hospital, Okinawa where she also assisted in the training of Japanese medical students. She completed Emergency Medicine residency at the University of Maryland Medical System in Baltimore and served as Chief resident. Dr McMullin is a member of the American College of Emergency Physicians

Cynthia R. Biron, RHD, EMT, MA

Ms Biron is chairperson of the Tallahassee Community College Dental Health Programs. In addition to her administrative duties as chairperson, she teaches clinical dental hygiene, dental hygiene theory, medical emergencies and Allied Health pharmacology. She also teaches continuing education courses throughout the United States for private practitioners and dental educators. Ms Biron has over 20 years of sound, hands-on experience in private practice, emergency medicine, and dental profession's education. She received an AS degree in Dental Hygiene from New Hampshire Technical Institute in 1973, a BA in Medical Technology and Human Biology from Notre Dame College in New Hampshire in 1982, a certification as an emergency medical technician from the University of Texas Health Science Center in 1991, and an MA in adult higher education from the University of Texas at San Antonio in 1992. Ms Biron has taught medical emergencies and pharmacology at several community colleges in the nation and the University of Texas Health Science Center at San Antonio. In addition to numerous journal and textbook contributions, Ms Biron is a bimonthly columnist for RDH magazine's "Medical Alert" column.

Harold L. Crossley, DDS, PhD

Dr Crossley is Professor Emeritus at the University of Maryland Dental School. A native of Rhode Island, Dr Crossley received a Bachelor of Science degree in Pharmacy from the University of Rhode Island in 1964. He later was awarded the Master of Science (1970) and Doctorate degrees (1972) in Pharmacology. The University of Maryland Dental School in Baltimore awarded Dr Crossley the DDS degree in 1980. The liaison between the classroom and his dental practice, which he mentored on a part-time basis in the Dental School Intramural Faculty Practice, produced a practical approach to understanding the pharmacology of drugs used in the dental office.

Dr Crossley has coauthored a number of articles and four books dealing with a variety of topics within the field of pharmacology. Other areas of expertise include the pharmacology of street drugs and chemical dependency. He serves on the Maryland State Dental Association's Well-Being Committee, was a member of the University Interdisciplinary Committee for Drug Abuse Education, and served on the Governor's Commission on Prescription Drug Abuse. He is an active member of Phi Kappa Phi, Omicron Kappa Upsilon Honorary Dental Society, the American College of Dentists, and International College of Dentists. He has been a consultant for the United States Drug Enforcement Administration and other law enforcement agencies since 1974. Drawing on this unique background, Dr Crossley has become nationally and internationally recognized as an expert on street drugs and chemical dependency as well as the clinical pharmacology of dental drugs.

PREFACE

The authors are gratified with the enthusiastic response that *Dental Office Medical Emergencies* has received since its release. As a result of reader feedback and newly published guidelines, this new edition represents the state of the art in emergency medical care for dental patients. The latest guidelines for cardiac emergencies, hemorrhagic events, and infection exposures are presented.

ACKNOWLEDGMENTS

The *Dental Office Medical Emergencies* manual exists in its present form as the result of the concerted efforts of the following individuals: Brad Bolinski, Director, Dentistry Division and Lynn D. Coppinger, Managing Editor.

In particular, the authors wish to thank Phylis L. Wynn for her contribution to the cover design. Special thanks also go to Seth C. Meiller and Rebecca C. Meiller for their assistance in library research and typing of the initial drafts, as well as to the authors' families and colleagues who supported them in their effort to design and complete the manual.

INTRODUCTION

All dentists would like to avoid the problems associated with managing dental office medical emergencies. As practitioners, we cannot be certain that these situations will not occur. It is hoped that with preparation, most if not all dental office emergencies can be avoided. The best management of medical problems is always prevention. This text seeks to provide information to the practicing dentist and dental office personnel, so that prevention and management of office emergencies are an integral part of the normal operational knowledge base. The philosophy of this handbook is:

> **P** reparedness of dental office personnel to take on the role of the first responder

> **R** ecognition of predisposing history/presenting signs and symptoms of an emergency

> **A** ction to stabilize, using basic life support techniques, and/or treat the patient

> **Y** ell for help by activating the Emergency Medical System (EMS) when necessary

The American Dental Association's publication on dental therapeutics describes the incidence of medical emergencies in the dental office. Most of the problems that the dentist encounters are not life-threatening, but any emergency can become serious if not properly managed. If the dentist and dental office personnel can identify the signs and symptoms of a developing potential office emergency, many emergencies can be aborted and treated within the dental office.

Occasionally, life-threatening office emergencies occur and it is incumbent upon the dentist to be well prepared, to not only evaluate, but to act to stabilize, activate EMS, and manage/refer these patients to an appropriate medical facility for more definitive emergency care.

* * * * * * * * * *

THIS TEXT IS DESIGNED TO FACILITATE DENTAL OFFICE MEDICAL EMERGENCY PROTOCOLS AND TO ASSIST THE DENTIST IN ADDRESSING ANY DEVELOPING DENTAL OFFICE EMERGENCY BY REINFORCING BASIC LIFE SUPPORT TECHNIQUES. THIS TEXT IS NOT DESIGNED TO INSTRUCT THE PRACTITIONER OR ANYONE IN THE OFFICE IN EXTENDED ADVANCED LIFE SUPPORT TECHNIQUES.

* * * * * * * * * *

It is the premise of the authors that the dentist should be able to identify a developing problem and determine the need for assistance from emergency medical personnel. During that brief but vital time period, stabilization procedures are always the most appropriate care. This text is designed to assist in establishing basic office protocols for stabilization of any such patient. If the office is properly prepared, this book would not be needed during the actual emergency, but the protocols will have been committed to memory and it will be available should memory fail, and a quick reference is needed. Often, stabilization of the patient results in appropriate and adequate treatment, eliminating the patient's need to be transported to a medical facility. Having a sound knowledge base, the dentist can make this determination.

Following this introduction, the text is divided into three sections for easy access of information. The first section describes office preparedness and addresses the development of protocol and training for management of any potential office emergency. Three subsections include patient evaluation, office equipment, and training of personnel.

The second section addresses specific dental office medical emergency protocols that are defined by symptom analysis. The subjects are tabbed to be separated into major categories associated with life-threatening office emergencies and include:

> 1) Loss of Consciousness,

> 2) Respiratory Distress,

> 3) Chest Pain,

> 4) Allergic / Drug Reactions,

> 5) Altered Sensations / Changes in Affect, and

> 6) Management of Acute Bleeding.

Within each of these major symptom groups are other symptom-recognition categories that will allow the practitioner easy access to specific likely medical conditions associated with the incident and action plans. Relatively rare office emergencies (eg, thyroid storm) and emergencies that originate over longer time periods (eg, diabetic acidosis) have been mentioned, but not covered as separate protocols.

The last section of the text addresses information on office protocols for occupational injuries, protocols for measurement of vital signs by the American Heart Association, discussion of automated external defibrillators, oxygen delivery systems, and other useful information in establishing appropriate office protocols.

SECTION ONE: OFFICE PREPAREDNESS

HISTORY AND PHYSICAL EXAMINATION

The best tool to reduce the risk of a medical emergency occurring in the dental office is the patient's history and record. The dentist should collect adequate information to establish a complete baseline history on all new patients and an adequate updated history on all recall or patients returning to the office. Subjects that must be covered include:

History and physical examination on all new patients

Baseline history	Allergies
Medications	Need for and results of medical consultation
Past/current medical conditions	Baseline vital signs – pulse, blood pressure, respirations, temperature

Having this information available in the patient record in a format that is easily accessible by trained dental office personnel, allows quick reference of baseline values should a medical emergency occur during the delivery of dental care.

In today's dental practice, some clinicians believe that patient care has become more complicated due to increased use of over-the-counter and prescription medications, as well as the increased complexity of medical diagnoses and management. Other clinicians believe that technological and medical care advances have actually simplified patient care. For the most part, patients seeking elective dental care are adequately managed medically. Patients often appear to have complications based on history, but may be quite stable. New patients and patients with dental emergencies require special attention on the part of the practitioner. It is incumbent upon the dentist to be able to adequately evaluate complete histories and the current medical status of patients, so patients can be assessed for any potential risk while undergoing dental procedures. Each dental office should design a history format that works best for them.

Obtaining the history is usually the first and often the most important interaction with any new patient and with any patient of record that is being re-evaluated after a period of time. Many techniques can be used when addressing sensitive or complicated medical information. Most commonly, the medical history addresses major medical problems in the form of a questionnaire; it follows a review-of-systems format in addressing other symptomatology, which might be present, but remains undiagnosed to-date. This style is often supplemented with a narrative description by the interviewer. Regardless of the technique used, all dental office personnel should be familiar with how to access the information and should have adequate medical knowledge to alert the dentist to any known pre-existing conditions.

A review of current medications must also be included. The review must include home remedies, nonprescription drugs, vitamins or dietary supplements, and medications not prescribed to the patient (available friends or relatives) but may have been used by the patient. Doses and frequency of use are important. Drugs that have known associations with some medical emergencies are listed with each protocol. It is not the intent of this manual to provide detailed drug information on every drug mentioned that has potential side effects or a specific incidence of adverse events or drug interactions. The reader should consult the latest edition of Lexi-Comp's *Drug Information Handbook for Dentistry* or any other drug information database to stay current with these concerns if such drugs are identified in a patient's history.

Certain drug classes are associated with potential dental office medical emergencies. Syncope can be caused by $alpha_1$-adrenergic receptor blockers (used to treat hypertension), nitroglycerin, some tricyclic antidepressants, and those antipsychotics which inhibit dopamine type 2 receptors and block $alpha_1$-adrenergic receptors (ie, clozapine). Orthostatic or postural hypotension can also be caused by medication in these drug classes. In addition, this condition has occurred in patients taking angiotensin-converting enzyme (ACE) inhibitors, calcium channel blockers, or beta-adrenergic receptor blockers for hypertension. Hypoglycemia is associated with the oral antidiabetic drugs. These associations are not always obvious, but the dentist should be attentive to the increased risk when patients are taking drugs in these therapeutic categories.

Allergies must be covered in some detail so the dentist is made aware of any known pre-existing allergies, either to environmental agents or medications. Medical reactions or toxicities in the dental office can result in serious life-threatening symptoms. Recognizing any predisposing history may allow the dentist to avoid these interactions or recognize them should they occur. Previous substance abuse might predispose the patient to drug reactions, and untoward medical response, during the delivery of dental care.

If the past history and general state of health, as well as the current physical evaluation, determines that a patient requires medical consultation, this should be noted in the patient's record. The reason for the consultation and the outcome should be clearly indicated in the record so the dentist is aware of the result of such consultation at each subsequent visit. This readiness may reduce risk.

As part of the normal physical examination that the dentist provides for each new patient and each recall patient, vital signs should be recorded (refer to Section Three). In most instances, these procedures are limited to measurements of pulse and blood pressure; however, in instances where any predisposing conditions might warrant or suggest more detailed evaluation, baseline respiratory rate and temperature might also be recorded. These data should be available and readily accessible in each patient's record so that, should an office emergency occur, the dental office personnel can compare the status during the emergency with the baseline data.

Elaborate schemes are available in oral medicine texts (see References and Recommended Readings section) that assign risk by a variety of classifications. One method is to use the American Society of Anesthesiologists classification scheme to evaluate whether a patient's pre-existing medical condition places them at high risk during the delivery of anesthesia. Another mechanism is to assign the risk of dental procedures based on an analysis of pre-existing medical conditions matched with the complexity of the planned dental procedure. This protocol takes into account the potential invasiveness of the dental procedure. Simple procedures in complicated patients may have low total risk, whereas complex procedures in simple patients may place the patient at significant risk for an office emergency. Each dental practitioner should design or adapt a patient analysis plan for their own office.

EQUIPMENT

The dental office should be adequately equipped to not only deliver routine care to each new patient and each returning patient, but also should be set up for appropriate management and stabilization of any potential office emergency. This requires that each patient and treatment area should be equipped with a minimum of a blood pressure cuff and a stethoscope. The office should also have available:

Appropriately-sized blood pressure cuffs

Tourniquets

Stethoscopes

First-aid kits

Emergency number call list

Emergency cabinet

Nasal cannula

Masks (nonrebreather and a bag-valve mask [Ambu®])

Oxygen tank (size E portable with low flow regulator); refer to Oxygen Delivery

Syringes (intramuscular: I.M. 3 cc disposable, subcutaneous: SubQ tuberculin)

Albuterol inhaler or solution/apparatus for nebulization

Automated external defibrillator (AED), if available; refer to AED

The emergency call list should be properly posted so office personnel need not search other operatories or the reception area for such information. Centrally-located emergency cabinets, which include tourniquets, emergency medical care drugs, instruments, and supplies, are essential.

DENTAL OFFICE EMERGENCY DRUGS

Protocols should be established for most office emergencies. Recognition and rapid diagnosis lead to appropriate management. Major drugs usually available in the emergency drug cabinet, discussed (regarding emergency use) in the Alphabetical Listing of Drugs section, are listed below and are described in more detail on the following pages.

Albuterol

Aluminum Chloride

Aminocaproic Acid

Ammonia Spirit, Aromatic

Aspirin

Cellulose (Oxidized / Regenerated)

Collagen (Absorbable)

Dexamethasone — (Alternative is Solu-Cortef® Mix-O-Vials for I.M.; has a longer shelf life)

Dextrose

Diazepam (Valium®)

Diphenhydramine (Benadryl®)

Epinephrine — (AnaKit® includes preloaded Tubex® syringes, which have measured dosing in increments)

Fibrin Sealant Kit

Flumazenil

Gelatin (Absorbable)

Glucagon Injectable

Glucose — (Emergency kit should also have oral carbohydrate source, such as Glutose 15™ oral gel and injectable glucagon)

Hydrocortisone — (Alternative is Solu-Cortef® Mix-O-Vials for I.M.; has a longer shelf life)

- Lorazepam
- Methylprednisolone (Solu-Medrol®)
- Microfibrillar Collagen (Absorbable)
- Morphine
- Naloxone (Narcan®)
- Nitroglycerin
- Oxygen
- Promethazine
- Thrombin (Topical)

Drug cabinet supplies should be in dose forms which the dentist is comfortable administering. Typical routes of administration could include oral (eg, diphenhydramine), inhalation (eg, albuterol), intramuscular/I.M. (eg, hydrocortisone), subcutaneous/SubQ (eg, epinephrine), or intravenous/I.V. (eg, epinephrine). Sublingual/S.L. injection can be substituted for some I.V. administrations in situations (ie, anaphylaxis) where a drug such as epinephrine may be life-saving. Oral mucosal absorption (eg, nitroglycerin) is also useful.

EMERGENCY CART SUPPLIES

I.V. Supplies
Fluids: 1 L (0.9% NS, 250 cc D_5W)
Tubing: (2) 60 gtt/cc I.V. tubings
Access: (2) each 20 gg, 22 gg angiocaths (1) - 24 gg
Alcohol wipes, gauze, tape, Tegaderm® and med lock hoop
(2) prefilled 3 cc syringes 0.9% NS

Syringes and Needles
(2) 1 cc TB/insulin syringe
(2-3) 3 cc syringes
(2) 5 cc syringes
Needles: 18, 22, 25 gauge

Respiratory Support
Airways: Adults large, medium, and small; Child - Peds Cart has infant size
(2) nasal cannulas
(1) 100% nonrebreather mask
(1) one-way valve mask (not in all carts - on order)
(1) Adult 100% Ambu® bag with mask

Miscellaneous
Ice pack
4 x 4s

STAFF TRAINING

It is imperative that all dental office personnel be trained to assist in routine patient care as well as potential office emergencies in an appropriate and timely manner. There should be an office plan in place with individual responsibilities and assignments established in the event of any office emergency. This plan should include assignment of essential duties during an office emergency. Simple codes can be used for communication so as not to alarm other patients.

Each dental office should design a plan that will work well in their facility with their personnel arrangement. A typical plan might include the dentist monitoring vital signs or treating the patient, while the dental assistant accesses the patient record for any baseline information. Another assistant should be collecting equipment, such as the emergency cart or first-aid equipment, to be chair-side for the dentist's use. The receptionist could be assigned the duty of calling emergency medical personnel, or being ready to make this call. Additional duties might include assisting with CPR or transporting and positioning the patient. Physical requirements for these activities may mandate that the dentist be the primary person to carry out these activities.

Regardless of the protocol designed for the individual dental office, it is imperative that each person in the office knows his or her duty, and to be trained in identifying some of the basic symptomatology described in this text. Often, emergencies occur when the dentist is either out of the room or working with another patient. This situation makes it incumbent on personnel who may be with the patient, to be able to quickly assess the need to alert the dentist for management of the potential emergency.

Office personnel, including the dentist, dental hygienists, and dental assistants, should all be trained in measurement of vital signs. Primarily, this includes measurement of pulse and evaluation of blood pressure. Proper technique for evaluating vital signs is necessary so information is accurate, and in the event of an emergency situation, ongoing measurements could be made by assisting personnel. The dentist should be able to provide this training to new employees, however, continuing education courses in proper technique are available.

Dental office personnel should all be trained in basic life support first-aid, although the dentist is ultimately in charge of delivering care to either patient or personnel. Each office member should be aware of basic principles for management of nonlife-threatening injuries. All office personnel should be trained in cardiopulmonary resuscitation (CPR) or basic life support (BLS).

Training courses are readily available through the American Heart Association and/or hospital facilities in most areas. Training should include not only basic initial training, but also renewal of skills should be a requirement for continued employment. One to two years is a reasonable time for updating such skills in cardiopulmonary resuscitation. Applicable state requirements or recommendations should be reviewed.

It is equally important that all dental office personnel understand the procedure for occupational exposures. Although this is part of emergency and first-aid care, the personnel should be aware of the protocol should either an infectious risk exposure occur or some other injury results in an occupational exposure of either an infectious or potentially toxic agent. Section Three describes the standard occupational protocol.

* * * * * * * * * *

It is the objective of this text to avoid discussion of advanced life support techniques such as those carried out by EMT and en route to the hospital emergency room. Many dentists have been trained in some aspects of advanced life support. It is the opinion of the authors that a dental office setting is not the place to attempt advanced life support without sufficient training, maintenance of skills, and the assistance of emergency medical personnel. The well-prepared dental office staff is CPR- and AED-certified.

Medicolegally, in most states, the dentist must be able to evaluate a patient historically and, at the very minimum, provide emergency first-aid care prior to the invitation to emergency medical personnel to take over in the event of a medical problem. In the event of a life-threatening office emergency, the dentist should feel comfortable with basic life support techniques and should be able to stabilize a patient to the point of waiting for the emergency medical transport to arrive. If no one is going to accompany the patient to the hospital, then a telephone call to the receiving hospital would be helpful to provide any historical information on the patient for the hospital records.

* * * * * * * * * *

MEASURING VITAL SIGNS

The vital signs are pulse, respiration, and blood pressure. Vital signs assess the stability of the patient and can alert you to problems that require immediate attention.

A **pulse rate** <50 beats per minute and a pulse rate >120 beats per minute are both considered serious. If a patient is unconscious, there is very little you can do to change the pulse rate. If the patient is conscious, then you can help. Talking to the patient, assuring him that you can help and that more help is on the way may prove to be significant. Having the patient answer you as you talk may help. As the patient relaxes and stays aware, rapid pulse rates will often decrease and low pulse rates will often increase. Sometimes, in emergency situations, simple reassuring conversation with the patient could change the pulse rate some 10 beats per minute.

A **respiration rate** >30 breaths per minute is considered to be a serious condition. Again, through conversation with the conscious patient, you can make a difference.

PULSE

Two factors, rate and character, must be determined when evaluating a patient's pulse. In terms of rate, you have to determine the number of beats per minute. This will provide you with the information necessary to decide if the patient's pulse rate is NORMAL, RAPID, or SLOW. Character considers the rhythm and force of the pulse. You will judge the pulse as being REGULAR or IRREGULAR in regard to rhythm and FULL or THREADY (weak) in regard to force.

The first thing you should do once you have found the patient's pulse is to make a quick judgment as to its rate. Simply determined if you believe the pulse rate to be in the normal range or if it is slow or rapid.

Next, you will determine the actual pulse rate. While you are doing this, notice if the beats are regular, regardless of the rate of the pulse. A rapid, regular beat is quite different in meaning from a rapid, irregular beat. At the same time, judge the force of the pulse. If it is strong and you have the impression that a wave of blood is passing under your fingertips, then judge the pulse as full. If you feel a weak pulse, causing you to believe that the flow is "thin", then judge the pulse as thready. Before you finish counting the pulse beats to find rate, you should be able to say if the pulse is rapid or slow, regular or irregular, and full or thready, based upon judgment. Some medications, such as beta-blockers, may slow the pulse. The patient may be aware of their typical pulse rate.

During the secondary survey, a wrist (radial) pulse is measured and is named for the radial artery found in the lateral portion of the forearm. If you cannot measure the radial pulse, determine pulse rate and characteristics by using the carotid pulse. If you find no pulse at the wrist, you must take a carotid pulse. **DO NOT start CPR based upon a radial pulse.**

Diagnostic Sign: Pulse

Observation	Possible Problem
Rapid, full	Panic attack, overexertion, heat stroke, high blood pressure, internal bleeding (early stages)
Rapid, thready	Shock, blood loss, heat exhaustion, diabetic coma, failing circulatory system
Slow, full	Stroke, skull fracture
No pulse	Cardiac arrest

Measuring Radial Pulse Rate

— Use the three middle fingers of your hand. Do not use your thumb to measure pulse rate.

— Place your fingertips on the palm side of the patient's hand, just above the crease between hand and wrist. Slide your fingers from this position toward the thumb side of the wrist (lateral side). Keeping the fingertip of the middle finger on the crease between wrist and hand will assure you of placing one fingertip over the site of the radial pulse.

— Apply moderate pressure to feel the pulse beats. If the pulse is weak, you may have to apply more pressure. Too much pressure can cause problems for blood flow. By having three fingers in contact with the patient's wrist and hand, you should be able to judge the pressure you are applying.

— Once you can feel pulsations, make a quick judgment as to rate. Rapid or slow?

— Count the number of beats for 15 seconds.

— While counting, judge rhythm and force.

— Multiply your count by 4 to determine the radial pulse rate in beats per minute.

The normal pulse rate for adults, when they are at rest, will fall between 60-80 beats per minute. In emergency situations, it is not unusual for this rate to be around 100 beats per minute. Consider >120 beats per minute and <50 beats per minute to be serious situations. Any rate >80 is rapid and any rate <60 is slow.

RESPIRATIONS

The rate and character of respiration are both considered. Rate of respiration is classified as NORMAL, RAPID, and SLOW. Character will include RHYTHM, DEPTH, SOUND, and EASE of the breathing.

A single respiration is the entire cycle of breathing in and out. While you are counting these cycles, note if the rhythm is regular or irregular. At the same time, decide if the depth of breathing is *normal, shallow,* or *deep.*

While measuring respiration rate, listen for any sounds that are not typically heard during respiration: Is there a snoring sound, gurgling, gasping, or bird-like crowing sounds?

Diagnostic Sign: Respirations

Observation	Possible Problem
Rapid, shallow	Shock, cardiac dysfunction, heat exhaustion, insulin shock, heart failure
Deep, gasping, labored	Airway obstruction, heart failure, heart attack, lung disease, chest injury, lung damage from heat, diabetic coma
Snoring	CVA/stroke, fractured skull, drug or alcohol
Crowing	Airway obstruction, airway injury due to heat
Gurgling	Airway obstruction, lung disease, lung injury due to heat
Coughing blood	Chest wound, fractured rib, punctured lung, internal injuries

Measuring Respiration Rate and Character

- Remain in the same position you assumed for measuring pulse. Keep your fingers on the patient's wrist as if you are still monitoring pulse rate.

- Watch the patient's chest movements and listen for sounds.

- Count the number of breaths (one breath = one inspiration and one expiration) the patient takes in 15 seconds. Multiply this number by 4 to obtain breaths per minute.

- While counting respirations, note rhythm, depth, sound, and ease of breathing.

If you have difficulty in establishing the rate of respiration, gently place your hand on the patient's chest, near the xiphoid process. This will allow you to feel each inspiration and expiration.

Normal respiration rates for adults at rest fall into a range of 12-20 breaths per minute, with most people having 12-15 breaths per minute as their normal range. Older adults tend to breathe more slowly than young adults. Infants can have a range from 35-50 breaths per minute. For adults, a rate >30 breaths per minute is serious. If the patient is a child from 1-5 years of age, a rate >44 breaths per minute is serious; a rate >36 breaths per minute is serious for children from 5-12 years of age.

BLOOD PRESSURE

Each time the lower chamber of the left side of the heart contracts, it forces blood out into circulation. The pressure created in the arteries by this blood is called the *systolic* blood pressure. When the lower left chamber of the heart is relaxed and refilling, the pressure in the arteries is called the *diastolic* blood pressure. The systolic pressure is reported first, as in "120 over 80."

Since you have no way of knowing the patient's normal blood pressure, one reading of blood pressure is not very meaningful. You will have to make several readings over a period of time while care is provided at the scene and during transport. Remember that changes in blood pressure are diagnostically significant.

Serious low blood pressure (hypotension) is generally considered to be <90 mm Hg, systolic. High blood pressure (hypertension) exists once the pressure rises >140/90. Keep in mind that many individuals in emergency situations will show a temporary rise in blood pressure. Anytime a patient's blood pressure drops to ≤90/60, it is possible that the patient is going into shock.

Table 1.

Classification and Management of Blood Pressure for Adults Aged 18 Years of Age or Older

BP Classification	Systolic BP (mm Hg)		Diastolic BP (mm Hg)	Medical Management*		
					Initial Drug Therapy	
				Lifestyle Modification	Without Compelling Indication	With Compelling Indications†
Normal	<120	and	<80	Encourage		
Prehypertension	120-139	or	80-89	Yes	No antihypertensive drug indicated	Drug(s) for the compelling indications‡
Stage 1 Hypertension	140-159	or	90-99	Yes	Thiazide-type diuretics for most; may consider ACE inhibitor, ARB, beta-blocker, CCB, or combination	Drug(s) for the compelling indications. Other antihypertensive drugs (diuretics, ACE inhibitor, ARB, beta-blocker, CCB) as needed
Stage 2 Hypertension	≥160	or	≥100	Yes	2-Drug combination for most (usually thiazide-type diuretic and ACE inhibitor or ARB or beta-blocker or CCB)#	Drug(s) for the compelling indications. Other antihypertensive drugs (diuretics, ACE inhibitor, ARB, beta-blocker, CCB) as needed

Abbreviations: ACE = angiotensin-converting enzyme; ARB = angiotensin-receptor blocker; BP = blood pressure; CCB = calcium channel blocker
*Treatment determined by highest BP category.
†See list in Table 2.
‡Treat patients with chronic kidney disease or diabetes to BP goal of <130/80 mm Hg.
#Initial combined therapy should be used cautiously in those at risk for orthostatic hypotension.
Adapted from Dalal S, The Seventh Report of the Joint National Committee on Prevention, Detection, Evaluation, and Treatment of High Blood Pressure (The JNC VII Guidelines), *Hypertension*, 2003, 42(6):1206-52.

Table 2.

Compelling Indications for Initiating Drugs of Certain Antihypertensive Class

1. **Ischemic heart disease:**
   a. Stable angina - beta-blocker is preferred. Long-acting calcium channel blockers are suggested as a second agent.
   b. Acute coronary syndrome - hypertension should be treated initially with beta-blocker and ACE inhibitor.
   c. Postmyocardial infarction patients - ACE inhibitors, beta-blockers, and aldosterone antagonists.

2. **Heart failure:**
   a. In asymptomatic individuals with left ventricular dysfunction, ACE inhibitors and beta-blockers are recommended.
   b. In symptomatic left ventricular dysfunction ACE inhibitors, beta-blockers, ARBs, aldosterone blockers, and loop diuretics are recommended.

3. **Diabetic with hypertension:**
   a. Combinations of two or more drugs are usually needed to lower blood pressure to a goal of <130/80 mm.
   b. Thiazide diuretics, beta-blockers, ACE inhibitors, ARBs, calcium channel blockers reduce cardiovascular disease/stroke incidence.
   c. ACE inhibitors/ARBs reduce progression of diabetic nephropathy/albuminuria.

4. **Chronic renal disease:**
   a. Defined as GFR <60 cc per minute or presence or albuminuria >300 mg/d or 200 mg albumin per gram of creatinine, needs aggressive treatment of hypertension to a target of <130/80 mm Hg. ACE inhibitors and ARBs reduce the progression of renal disease in both diabetic and nondiabetic renal disease.
   b. Increase in creatinine up to 35% above baseline with an ACE inhibitor/ARBs is acceptable unless hyperkalemia develops. In patients with GFR <30 cc/minute (creatinine 2.5-3 mg/dL) increasing doses of loop diuretics in combination with other class of drugs is usually necessary.

5. **Cerebral vascular disease:**
   a. Risks and benefits of acute lowering of blood pressure during acute CVA are still unclear.
   b. Recurrent stroke rates are lowered by ACE Inhibitors and thiazide-type diuretics.

6. **Minority populations:**
   a. In African-American patients there is a somewhat reduced blood pressure response to monotherapy to beta-blockers, ACE inhibitors and ARBs compared to diuretics or calcium channel blockers. The differential responses are largely eliminated by drug combinations that include adequate doses of a diuretic.
   b. ACE inhibitors induce angioedema two to four times more often in African-Americans.

7. **Hypertension in women:**
   a. Monitor blood pressure regularly in women on oral contraceptives due to increased risk of hypertension.
   b. Hypertensive women who get pregnant should be monitored very closely. Methyldopa, vasodilators, and some beta-blockers and calcium channel blockers are preferred antihypertensives during pregnancy for the safety of the fetus. ACE inhibitors/ARBs are contraindicated in pregnancy and in women likely to become pregnant.

Table 3.

Dental Management and BP Levels

BP <140/90 mmHg proceed with regular dental care and advise lifestyle changes for the patients with prehypertension.

BP 140-159/90-99 Regular dental care, physician consult and lifestyle changes.

BP >160/100, repeat BP after 5 minutes; noninvasive care only, refer to MD.

BP >220/120 refer to MD and/or nearest ER.

Table 4.

Components of Cardiovascular Risk Stratification in Patients With Hypertension

Major Risk Factors

    Smoking

    Dyslipidemia

    Diabetes mellitus

    Age >60 years

    Sex (men and postmenopausal women)

    Family history of cardiovascular disease: women <65 years of age or men <55 years of age

Target Organ Damage/Clinical Cardiovascular Disease

    Heart diseases

    Left ventricular hypertrophy

    Angina/prior myocardial infarction

    Prior coronary revascularization

    Heart failure

    Stroke or transient ischemic attack

    Nephropathy

    Peripheral arterial disease

    Retinopathy

DETERMINING BLOOD PRESSURE BY AUSCULTATION

Begin by placing the ends of the stethoscope arms in your ears. With your fingertips, palpate the brachial artery at the crease of the elbow. Position the diaphragm or bell of the stethoscope directly over the brachial pulse site. With the bulb valve closed, inflate the cuff. As you do so, you will be able to hear pulse sounds. Inflate the cuff, watching the gauge. At a certain point, you will no longer hear the brachial pulse. Continue to inflate the cuff until the gauge reads 20 mm Hg higher than the point where the pulse sound disappeared.

Slowly release air from the cuff by opening the bulb valve, allowing the pressure to fall smoothly at the rate of 2-3 mm Hg per second.

Listen for the start of clicking or tapping sounds. When you hear the beginning of these sounds, note the reading on the gauge. This is the systolic pressure. Continue to deflate the cuff, listening for when these distinctive sounds fade (not when they disappear). When the sounds turn to dull, muffled thuds, the reading on the gauge is the diastolic pressure. After obtaining the diastolic pressure, let the cuff deflate. If you are not certain of a reading, repeat the procedure. You should use the other arm, or wait one minute before reinflating the cuff. Otherwise, you will tend to obtain an erroneously high reading.

REMEMBER: Blood pressure must be measured while a person is seated or lying down. Do **NOT** move a patient simply to determine blood pressure. To do so may aggravate existing injuries. Always try to keep the cuff at heart level. If the patient is sitting up, support his arm (eg, on the arm of a chair) or hold the patient's arm during the entire procedure.

CPR & BASIC LIFE SUPPORT

BLS

Basic life support (BLS) is a level of medical care which is used for patients with life-threatening illness or injury until the patient can be given full medical care. It can be provided by trained medical personnel, including emergency medical technicians, and by laypersons who have received BLS training. BLS is generally used in the pre-hospital setting, and can be provided without medical equipment.

Many countries have guidelines on how to provide basic life support (BLS) which are formulated by professional medical bodies in those countries. The guidelines outline algorithms for the management of a number of conditions, such as Cardiac arrest, choking and drowning.

BLS generally does not include the use of drugs or invasive skills, and can be contrasted with the provision of Advanced Life Support (ALS). Most laypersons can master BLS skills after attending a short course. Firefighters and police officers are often required to be BLS certified. BLS is also immensely useful for many other professions, such as day care providers, teachers and security personnel.

CPR provided in the field buys time for higher medical responders to arrive and provide ALS care. For this reason it is essential that any person starting CPR also obtains ALS support by calling for help via radio using agency policies and procedures and/or using an appropriate emergency telephone number.

An important advance in providing BLS is the availability of the automated external defibrillator or AED, which can be used to defibrillation or delivery. This improves survival outcomes in cardiac arrest cases.

BLS, in the United States, is generally identified with Emergency Medical Technicians-Basic (EMT-B). However, the American Heart Association's BLS protocol is designed for use by lay people, first responders, EMT-B, and to some extent, higher medical functions. It covers cardiac arrest, respiratory arrest, drowning, and foreign body airway obstruction (FBAO, or choking). EMT-B is the highest level of healthcare provider that is limited to the BLS protocol; higher medical functions use some or all of the Advanced Life Support (ALS) protocols, in addition to BLS protocols.

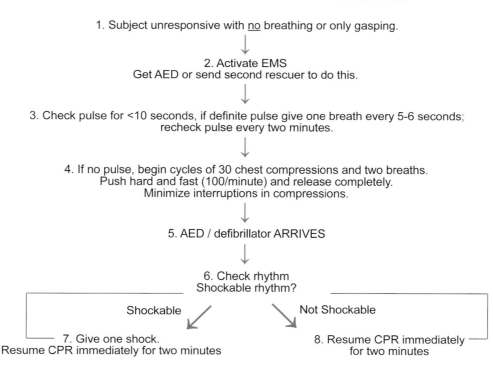

2010 ADULT BLS HEALTHCARE PROVIDER ALGORITHM

1. Subject unresponsive with <u>no</u> breathing or only gasping.

2. Activate EMS
Get AED or send second rescuer to do this.

3. Check pulse for <10 seconds, if definite pulse give one breath every 5-6 seconds; recheck pulse every two minutes.

4. If no pulse, begin cycles of 30 chest compressions and two breaths. Push hard and fast (100/minute) and release completely. Minimize interruptions in compressions.

5. AED / defibrillator ARRIVES

6. Check rhythm
Shockable rhythm?

Shockable   Not Shockable

7. Give one shock.
Resume CPR immediately for two minutes

8. Resume CPR immediately for two minutes

Check rhythm every two minutes.
Continue until ALS providers take over or victim starts to move.

The algorithm for providing basic life support to adults in the USA was published in 2010 in the journal *Circulation* by the American Heart Association (AHA)[1,2].

This section is an overview of the 2010 BLS standards. It is meant to be a helpful guide in an emergency and to reinforce procedures learned in a full CPR certification course. Considering the major 2010 changes in BLS and CPR, all personnel are urged to be recertified as soon as possible using the new order of action "CAB" – namely Compressions, Airway, and finally Breathing.

The AHA uses four-link "Chain of Survival" to illustrate the steps needed to resuscitate a collapsed victim:

1. Early recognition of the emergency and activation of emergency medical services

2. Early bystander CPR, so as not to delay treatment until arrival of EMS

3. Early use of a defibrillator

4. Early advanced life support and postresuscitation care

Bystanders with training in BLS can perform the first 3 of the 4 steps.

ADULT BLS SEQUENCE

- Ensure that the scene is safe.

- Assess the victim's level of consciousness by asking loudly "are you okay?" and by checking for the victim's responsiveness to pain.

- Activate the local EMS system by instructing someone to call 911. If an AED is available, it should be retrieved and prepared.

- If the patient is breathing normally, he should be placed in the recovery position and monitored and transported; do not continue the BLS sequence.

- If the patient is not breathing or not breathing normally (ie. only gasping) and/or the arrest was witnessed, then CPR until an AED arrives is the treatment of choice.

- Assess for the presence of a pulse at the carotid artery for no more than 10 seconds. If a pulse is definitely detected, the patient should continue to receive artificial ventilations at a rate of 1 breath every 5-6 seconds and be transported immediately. Otherwise, begin CPR: cycles of 30 compressions first, then 2 breaths.

- Compressions should be done at a rate of at least 100/minute and a depth of at least 2 inches, the chest should be allowed to completely recoil after each compression, and interruptions to compressions should be minimized.

- If the victim has no suspected cervical trauma, open the airway using the head-tilt/chin-lift maneuver; if the victim has suspected trauma, the airway should be opened with the jaw-thrust technique. If the jaw-thrust is ineffective at opening/maintaining the airway, the head-tilt/chin-lift should be performed.

- Deliver each rescue breath over 1 second and give sufficient tidal volume to produce visible chest rise while avoiding excessive ventilation. If ventilation is unsuccessful, reposition the airway and try again. If ventilation is still unsuccessful and the victim is unconscious, it is possible that they have a foreign body in their airway.

- When using an advanced airway (ie. endotracheal tube, Combitube, laryngeal mask airway [LMA]) during 2-person CPR, give one breath every 6-8 seconds and do not pause compressions to give breaths.

- After 5 cycles/2 minutes of CPR, the BLS protocol should be repeated from the beginning by doing a pulse check for no more than 10 seconds and resuming compressions. As soon as an AED is available, CPR should be interrupted to attach, activate, and defibrillate if indicated. Immediately resume CPR after shock/assessment for 5 cycles/2 minutes and check the rhythm every 2 minutes.

- BLS protocols continue until (1) the patient regains a pulse or starts to move, (2) the rescuer is relieved by another rescuer of equivalent or higher training, (3) the rescuer is too physically tired to continue CPR, or (4) the patient is pronounced dead by a medical doctor.

- The CPR cycle is often abbreviated as 30:2 (30 compressions, 2 ventilations or breaths). Note CPR for infants and children uses a 15:2 cycle when two rescuers are performing CPR (but still uses a 30:2 if there is only one rescuer).

DROWNING

- Rescuers should provide CPR as soon as an unresponsive victim is removed from the water. In particular, rescue breathing is important in this situation.

- A lone rescuer should give 5 cycles of CPR before leaving the victim to call emergency medical services. A cycle of CPR consists of giving 30 chest compressions and 2 breaths to the victim.

Since the primary cause of cardiac arrest and death in drowning and choking victims is hypoxia, it is more important to provide rescue breathing as quickly as possible in these situations, whereas for victims of VF cardiac arrest, chest compressions and defibrillation are more important.

HYPOTHERMIA

- In unresponsive victims with no normal breathing, CPR should be initiated if there is no definite pulse felt after 10 seconds. Of note, breathing and pulse may be significantly slowed which will make assessment more difficult.

- If cardiac arrest is confirmed, CPR should be started immediately. Wet clothes should be removed, and the victim should be insulated from wind. CPR should be continued until the victim is assessed by advanced care providers.

FOREIGN BODY AIRWAY OBSTRUCTION (CHOKING)

- Rescuers should intervene in victims who show signs of severe airway obstruction, such as a silent cough, cyanosis, inability to speak or breathe, or unresponsiveness.

- If a victim is coughing forcefully, rescuers should not interfere with this process.

- If a victim shows signs of severe airway obstruction, abdominal thrusts should be applied in rapid sequence until the obstruction is relieved. If this is not effective, chest thrusts can also be used. Chest thrusts can also be used in obese victims or victims in late pregnancy. Abdominal thrusts should not be used in infants under 1 year of age due to risk of causing injury.

- If a victim becomes unresponsive, he should be lowered to the ground, and the rescuer should call EMS and initiate CPR (without doing pulse check). When the airway is opened during CPR, the rescuer should look into the mouth for an object causing obstruction, and remove it if it is evident.

These guidelines differ from previous versions in a number of ways:

- They allow the rescuer to diagnose cardiac arrest if the victim is unresponsive and not breathing normally.

- "Look, Listen, and Feel" for breathing has been removed from the sequence.

- Compressions are now done before rescue breaths.

- There is increased focus on quality compressions and avoiding excessive ventilations.

- Less importance is placed on pulse checks.

These changes were introduced to simplify the algorithm, to allow for faster decision making and to maximise the time spent giving chest compressions; this is because interruptions in chest compressions have been shown to reduce the chance of survival.[5] It is also acknowledged that rescuers may either be unable, or unwilling, to give effective rescue breaths; in this situation, continuing chest compressions alone is advised, although this is only effective for about 5 minutes[6].

REFERENCES

1. "Circulation," http://circ.ahajournals.org/cgi/content/full/122/18_suppl_3/S640.

2. 2010 American Heart Association Guidelines for Cardiopulmonary Resuscitation and Emergency Cardiovascular Care Science, Circulation, 2010, 122:S640-S656.

3. Resuscitation Council (UK) Adult Basic Life Support (2005).

4. European Resuscitation Council guidelines and CoSTR documents.

5. Eftestol T, Sunde K, and Steen PA, "Effects of interrupting precordial compressions on the calculated probability of defibrillation success during out-of-hospital cardiac arrest," Circulation, 2002,105:2270-3.

6. Hallstrom A, Cobb L, Johnson E, et al, "Cardiopulmonary resuscitation by chest compression alone or with mouth-to-mouth ventilation," N Engl J Med, 2000, 342:1546-53.

7. Nozioni primo soccorso BLS (Italian), PDF document (12p, 912 Kb)

AUTOMATED EXTERNAL DEFIBRILLATOR (AED)

As it has been stressed throughout this manual, dental office medical emergencies are usually best managed with basic life support (BLS) techniques and, following accurate recognition of the signs and symptoms, a call for EMS if appropriate. In the event that a potentially irreversible cardiac incident occurs that places the patient at risk for cardiac arrest, the dentist must be aware of the signs and symptoms of this life-threatening condition. Basic life support, as always, is the framework from which other actions must be taken. The automated external defibrillators (AED) have been available for nearly a decade. However, their recent popularity has been enhanced by the endorsement of the American Heart Association for its use by emergency transport vehicles and the lay person use of these devices in airplanes and other locations when medical personnel may not be readily available as part of an EMS response team. At present, there are no specific guidelines for use of AEDs or defibrillation in the dental office. The well-prepared dental office staff is, of course, CPR and AED-certified as part of the latest BLS standards. The American Dental Association endorses these standards. Florida currently mandates AEDs for all dental offices and other states are considering similar requirements.

Cardiac arrest is strictly defined as ventricular asystole, a total absence of ventricular contraction resulting in a stand-still of the heart and eventually death. In practical use, however, cardiac arrest includes several potentially reversible stages which, if recognized, can be treated with basic life support techniques supplemented with defibrillation and early EMS intervention. The key steps in addressing a cardiac arrest situation are: Early access: Recognition of the signs and symptoms, leading to basic life support initiation and activation of the EMS system; CPR as part of the BLS system begun within the first few moments following the likely cardiac arrest; early defibrillation; and rapid transport by EMS to the hospital.

In instances when ventricular tachycardia (VT) or ventricular fibrillation (VF) are the contributing conditions of cardiac arrest, defibrillation can enhance the potential for successful resuscitation of the patient. Defibrillation must be done within the first few minutes after sudden cardiac arrest in order to maximize the patient's chance for resuscitation. Resuscitation is the return of the patient's pulse and breathing. If VF is not treated promptly, the electrical activity in the heart will gradually stop. At this point, the heart cannot respond to a defibrillation shock. If an AED is not immediately available, CPR can help delay brain damage and prolong heart activity so that it can be treated with defibrillation. Although CPR may be an important component in resuscitating the patient, CPR alone will not resuscitate the patient! VF can be successfully treated in many cases if defibrillation is delivered within the first few critical minutes after sudden cardiac arrest. For every minute of delay in defibrillating the heart of an SCA victim, the chances of survival decrease by about 10 percent!* After 10 minutes, successful resuscitation is very rare. Dysrhythmias, if left untreated, will result in ventricular asystole and death. In the past, advanced cardiac life support teams at the hospital or associated with the EMS arrival team on site have been the sole determinants of the need for and use of defibrillation. AEDs are now readily available for use by nonmedical personnel and have a variety of safety mechanisms to ensure that they are not inappropriately used. In the dental office, it is not likely that a cardiac arrest situation will go unwitnessed. Therefore, activating basic life support, CPR, and defibrillation would have the greatest potential for success. Although useful in assisting with perfusion, it must be remembered that BLS and CPR alone require EMS follow-up and transport to the hospital.

AEDs are available from a variety of companies and are generally supplied with options including a fully automatic state (one that does not require operator interpretation of signs or symptoms of the data), various printout mechanisms to indicate the cardiac rhythm that is being accessed automatically by the machine, voice prompters and recorders, and a semi-automatic state (which allows the interpretation of data given by the machine to the operator prior to defibrillation). In the fully automatic state, defibrillation is applied by the machine to the victim after proper placement of the electrodes as determined by the presence of specific dysrhythmias (VF or VT) during the cardiac arrest state. Readers are referred to the various on-line, internet information sources for selection of one of the many AEDs on the market. Guidelines for utilization of AEDs in the dental office are currently under evaluation in numerous states and Florida currently requires their availability.

Adapted from Link MS, Atkins DL, Passman RS, et al, "Electrical Therapies: Automated External Defibrillators, Defibrillation, Cardioversion, and Pacing," 2010 American Heart Association Guidelines for Cardiopulmonary Resuscitation and Emergency Cardiovascular Care, *Circulation*, 2010, 122:S706-S719, doi: 10.1161/CIRCULATIONAHA. 110.970954.

EMERGENCY DRUG MONOGRAPHS

ALBUTEROL

Therapeutic Category Beta$_2$-Adrenergic Agonist

Use Bronchodilator in reversible airway obstruction due to asthma or COPD; prevention of exercise-induced bronchospasm in patients ≥12 years of age

Emergency Dosage Bronchospasm: Metered-dose inhaler (MDI): 2-4 puffs initially; may be repeated in 10-20 minutes

Usual Dosage: Oral:

Children:

2-6 years: 0.1-0.2 mg/kg/dose 3 times/day; maximum dose not to exceed 12 mg/day (divided doses)

6-12 years: 2 mg/dose 3-4 times/day; maximum dose not to exceed 24 mg/day (divided doses)

Children >12 years and Adults: 2-4 mg/dose 3-4 times/day; maximum dose not to exceed 32 mg/day (divided doses)

Elderly: 2 mg 3-4 times/day; maximum: 8 mg 4 times/day

Inhalation metered-dose inhaler (MDI): 90 mcg/spray:

Children <12 years: 1-2 inhalations 4 times/day using a tube spacer

Children ≥12 years and Adults: 1-2 inhalations every 4-6 hours; maximum: 12 inhalations/day

Exercise-induced bronchospasm: 2 inhalations 15 minutes before exercising

Inhalation: Nebulization: 2.5 mg = 0.5 mL of the 0.5% inhalation solution to be diluted in 1-2.5 mL of NS or 0.01-0.05 mL/kg of 0.5% solution every 4-6 hours; intensive care patients may require more frequent administration; minimum dose: 0.1 mL; maximum dose: 1 mL diluted in 1-2 mL normal saline

<5 years: 1.25-2.5 mg every 4-6 hours as needed

>5 years: 2.5-5 mg every 4-6 hours as needed

Mechanism of Action Relaxes bronchial smooth muscle by action on beta$_2$-adrenergic receptors with little effect on heart rate

ALUMINUM CHLORIDE

Therapeutic Category Astringent; Hemostatic Agent

Use Hemostatic; gingival retraction; to control bleeding created during a dental procedure

Mechanism of Action Precipitates tissue and blood proteins causing a mechanical obstruction to hemorrhage from injured blood vessels

AMINOCAPROIC ACID

Therapeutic Category Antifibrinolytic Agent; Antihemophilic Agent; Hemostatic Agent; Lysine Analog

Use Treatment of excessive bleeding from fibrinolysis

Usual Dosage

Acute bleeding syndrome:

Children (unlabeled use): Oral, I.V.: 100-200 mg/kg during the first hour, followed by continuous infusion at 33.3 mg/kg/hour or 100 mg/kg (oral or I.V.) every 6 hours

Adults: Oral, I.V.: 4-5 g during the first hour, followed by 1 g/hour for 8 hours or until bleeding controlled (maximum daily dose: 30 g)

Control bleeding in thrombocytopenia (unlabeled use): Adults:

Initial: I.V.: 100 mg/kg over 30-60 minutes

Maintenance: Oral: 1-3 g every 6 hours

Control oral bleeding in congenital and acquired coagulation disorder (unlabeled use): Adults: Oral: 50-60 mg/kg every 4 hours

Traumatic hyphema (unlabeled use): Children and Adults: Oral: 100 mg/kg/dose every 4 hours (maximum daily dose: 30 g)

Prevention of dental procedure bleeding in patients on oral anticoagulant therapy (unlabeled use): Oral rinse: Hold 4 g/10 mL in mouth for 2 minutes then spit out. Repeat every 6 hours for 2 days after procedure (Souto, 1996). Concentration and frequency may vary by institution and product availability

Dosing adjustment in renal impairment: May accumulate in patients with decreased renal function.

Mechanism of Action Competitively inhibits activation of plasminogen to plasmin, also, a lesser antiplasmin effect

AMMONIA SPIRIT, AROMATIC

Therapeutic Category Respiratory Stimulant

Use Respiratory and circulatory stimulant, treatment of fainting

Usual Dosage Used as "smelling salts" to treat or prevent fainting

ASPIRIN

Therapeutic Category Antiplatelet Agent; Salicylate

Use

Dental: Treatment of postoperative pain

Medical: Treatment of mild-to-moderate pain, inflammation, and fever; prevention and treatment of myocardial infarction (MI), acute ischemic stroke, and transient ischemic episodes; management of rheumatoid arthritis, rheumatic fever, osteoarthritis, and gout (high dose); adjunctive therapy in revascularization procedures (coronary artery bypass graft [CABG], percutaneous transluminal coronary angioplasty [PTCA], carotid endarterectomy), stent implantation.

Usual Dosage

Analgesic: Oral:

Children: 10-15 mg/kg/dose every 4-6 hours, up to a total of 4 g/day

Adults: 325-650 mg (1-2 tablets) every 4-6 hours, up to 4 g/day

Mechanism of Action Irreversibly inhibits cyclooxygenase-1 and 2 (COX-1 and 2) enzymes, via acetylation, which results in decreased formation of prostaglandin precursors; irreversibly inhibits formation of prostaglandin derivative, thromboxane A$_2$, via acetylation of platelet cyclooxygenase, thus inhibiting platelet aggregation; has antipyretic, analgesic, and anti-inflammatory properties

CELLULOSE (Oxidized / Regenerated)

Therapeutic Category Hemostatic Agent

Use To control bleeding created during a dental procedure

Usual Dosage Minimal amounts of the fabric strip are laid on the bleeding site or held firmly against the tissues until hemostasis occurs; remove excess material

Mechanism of Action Cellulose, oxidized regenerated is saturated with blood at the bleeding site and swells into a brownish or black gelatinous mass which aids in the formation of a clot. When used in small amounts, it is absorbed from the sites of implantation with little or no tissue reaction. In addition to providing hemostasis, oxidized regenerated cellulose also has been shown in vitro to have bactericidal properties.

COLLAGEN (Absorbable)

Therapeutic Category Hemostatic Agent

Use To control bleeding created during dental surgery

Usual Dosage Children and Adults: A sufficiently large dressing should be selected so as to completely cover the oral wound

Mechanism of Action The highly porous sponge structure absorbs blood and wound exudate. The collagen component causes aggregation of platelets which bind to collagen fibrils. The aggregated platelets degranulate, releasing coagulation factors that promote the formation of fibrin.

DEXAMETHASONE

Therapeutic Category Anti-inflammatory Agent; Antiemetic; Corticosteroid, Inhalant (Oral)

Use
Dental: Treatment of a variety of oral diseases of allergic, inflammatory or autoimmune origin
Medical: Systemically and locally for chronic swelling, allergic, hematologic, neoplastic, and autoimmune diseases; may be used in management of cerebral edema, septic shock, as a diagnostic agent, antiemetic

Emergency Dosage Moderate to severe anaphylaxis, to prevent late-phase recurrence of symptoms: 4 mg I.V.

Usual Dosage
Children: Anti-inflammatory immunosuppressant: Oral, I.M., I.V. (injections should be given as sodium phosphate): 0.08-0.3 mg/kg/day or 2.5-10 mg/m2/day in divided doses every 6-12 hours
Adults: Anti-inflammatory:
Oral, I.M., I.V. (injections should be given as sodium phosphate): 0.5-9 mg/day in divided doses every 6-12 hours
I.M. (as acetate): 8-16 mg; may repeat in 1-3 weeks
Intralesional (as acetate): 0.8-1.6 mg
Topical: Apply a thin film to affected area once or twice daily

Mechanism of Action Decreases inflammation by suppression of migration of polymorphonuclear leukocytes and reversal of increased capillary permeability; suppresses normal immune response

DEXTROSE

Therapeutic Category Antidote, Hypoglycemia; Intravenous Nutritional Therapy

Use Oral: Treatment of hypoglycemia
5% and 10% solutions: Peripheral infusion to provide calories and fluid replacement
25% (hypertonic) solution: Treatment of acute symptomatic episodes of hypoglycemia in infants and children to restore depressed blood glucose levels; adjunctive treatment of hyperkalemia when combined with insulin
50% (hypertonic) solution: Treatment of insulin-induced hypoglycemia (hyperinsulinemia or insulin shock) and adjunctive treatment of hyperkalemia in adolescents and adults
≥10% solutions: Infusion after admixture with amino acids for nutritional support

Usual Dosage
Hypoglycemia: Doses may be repeated in severe cases
I.V.:
Infants ≤6 months: 0.25-0.5 g/kg/dose (1-2 mL/kg/dose of 25% solution); maximum: 25 g/dose
Infants >6 months and Children: 0.5-1 g/kg/dose (2-4 mL/kg/dose of 25% solution); maximum: 25 g/dose
Adolescents and Adults: 10-25 g (40-100 mL of 25% solution or 20-50 mL of 50% solution)
Oral: Children >2 years and Adults: 10-20 g as single dose; repeat in 10 minutes if necessary
Treatment of hyperkalemia: I.V. (in combination with insulin):
Infants and Children: 0.5-1 g/kg (using 25% or 50% solution) combined with regular insulin 1 unit for every 4-5 g dextrose given; infuse over 2 hours (infusions as short as 30 minutes have been recommended); repeat as needed
Adolescents and Adults: 25-50 g dextrose (250-500 mL D_{10}W) combined with 10 units regular insulin administered over 30-60 minutes; repeat as needed or as an alternative 25 g dextrose (50 mL D_{50}W) combined with 5-10 units regular insulin infused over 5 minutes; repeat as needed
Note: More rapid infusions (<30 minutes) may be associated with hyperglycemia and hyperosmolality and will exacerbate

hyperkalemia; avoid use in patients who are already hyperglycemic

Mechanism of Action Decreases inflammation by suppression of migration of polymorphonuclear leukocytes and reversal of increased capillary permeability; suppresses normal immune response

DIAZEPAM

Therapeutic Category Antianxiety Agent; Anticonvulsant, Benzodiazepine

Use
Dental: Oral medication for preoperative dental anxiety; sedative component in I.V. conscious sedation in oral surgery patients; skeletal muscle relaxant
Medical: In medicine, management of general anxiety disorders, panic disorders, and provide preoperative sedation, light anesthesia, and amnesia; treatment of status epilepticus, alcohol withdrawal symptoms; used as a skeletal muscle relaxant

Emergency Dosage I.V. push: 5-10 mg, not to exceed 5 mg minute

Usual Dosage
Children: Oral:
Conscious sedation for procedures: 0.2-0.3 mg/kg (maximum: 10 mg) 45-60 minutes prior to procedure
Sedation or muscle relaxation or anxiety: 0.12-0.8 mg/kg/day in divided doses every 6-8 hours the day before the procedure
Adults:
Oral: Preop sedation/antianxiety: 2-10 mg 2 times/day the day before the procedure; 2-10 mg morning of procedure if needed
I.V.: Conscious sedation: 5-15 mg titrated slowly to effect

Mechanism of Action Depresses all levels of the CNS, including the limbic and reticular formation, probably through the increased action of gamma-aminobutyric acid (GABA), which is a major inhibitory neurotransmitter in the brain

DIPHENHYDRAMINE HYDROCHLORIDE

Therapeutic Category Histamine H1 Antagonist; Histamine H1 Antagonist, First Generation

Use
Dental: Symptomatic relief of nasal mucosal congestion; symptomatic relief of oral erosions (systemic diphenhydramine used topically) including aphthous stomatitis
Medical: Can be used for mild nighttime sedation; prevention of motion sickness and as an antitussive; has antinauseant and topical anesthetic properties; treatment of phenothiazine-induced dystonic reactions

Usual Dosage Oral: Adults: 25-50 mg every 6-8 hours

Mechanism of Action Competes with histamine for H_1-receptor sites on effector cells in the gastrointestinal tract, blood vessels, and respiratory tract

EPINEPHRINE

Therapeutic Category Alpha/Beta Agonist

Use Dental: Emergency drug for treatment of anaphylactic reactions; used as vasoconstrictor to prolong local anesthesia

Emergency Dosage Anaphylactic shock, urticaria/pruritus: I.M., SubQ.: 0.3-0.5 mL of 1:1000 solution

Note: I.V. administration is generally not utilized unless cardiac monitoring is available and is used only in severe reactions (true anaphylaxis): 0.1 mg (1:10,000 solution) I.V. over 5 minutes

Usual Dosage Hypersensitivity reaction:
Children: I.M., SubQ: 0.01 mg/kg (0.01 mL/kg of 1:1000 solution) (maximum single dose: 0.5 mg) every 5-20 minutes; larger

I.M. or SubQ doses, use of I.V. route, or continuous infusion may be needed for severe anaphylactic reactions

Adults: I.M., SubQ.:0.3-0.5 mg (1:1000 solution) every 15-20 minutes if condition requires

Mechanism of Action Stimulates alpha-, beta$_1$-, and beta$_2$-adrenergic receptors resulting in relaxation of smooth muscle of the bronchial tree, cardiac stimulation, and dilation of skeletal muscle vasculature; small doses can cause vasodilation via beta$_2$-vascular receptors; large doses may produce constriction of skeletal and vascular smooth muscle; decreases production of aqueous humor and increases aqueous outflow; dilates the pupil by contracting the dilator muscle

FIBRIN SEALANT KIT

Therapeutic Category Hemostatic Agent
Use

Evicel™: Adjunct to hemostasis in liver or vascular surgery when control of bleeding by conventional surgical techniques is ineffective or impractical

Tisseel® VH: Adjunct to hemostasis in cardiopulmonary bypass surgery and splenic injury (due to blunt or penetrating trauma to the abdomen) when the control of bleeding by conventional surgical techniques is ineffective or impractical; adjunctive sealant for closure of colostomies; hemostatic agent in heparinized patients undergoing cardiopulmonary bypass

Usual Dosage Adjunct to hemostasis: Apply topically; actual dose is based on size of surface to be covered:

Evicel™: Children and Adults: Spray or drop onto surface of bleeding tissue in short bursts (0.1-0.2 mL); if hemostatic effect is not complete, apply a second layer. To cover a layer of 1 mm thickness:

Maximum area to be sealed: 20 cm^2
Required size of Evicel™ kit: 2 mL
Maximum area to be sealed: 40 cm^2
Required size of Evicel™ kit: 4 mL
Maximum area to be sealed: 100 cm^2
Required size of Evicel™ kit: 10 mL

Tisseel® VH: Adults: Apply in thin layers to avoid excess formation of granulation tissue and slow absorption of the sealant. Following application, hold the sealed parts in the desired position for 3-5 minutes. To prevent sealant from adhering to gloves or surgical instruments, wet them with saline prior to contact.

Maximum area to be sealed: 8 cm^2
Required package size of Tisseel® VH: 2 mL
Maximum area to be sealed: 16 cm^2
Required package size of Tisseel® VH: 4 mL
Maximum area to be sealed: 40 cm^2
Required package size of Tisseel® VH: 10 mL

Mechanism of Action Formation of a biodegradable adhesive is done by duplicating the last step of the coagulation cascade, the formation of fibrin from fibrinogen. Fibrinogen is the main component of the sealant solution. The solution also contains thrombin, which transforms fibrinogen from the sealer protein solution into fibrin, and fibrinolysis inhibitor (aprotinin), which prevents the premature degradation of fibrin. When mixed as directed, a viscous solution forms that sets into an elastic coagulum.

FLUMAZENIL

Therapeutic Category Antidote
Use Benzodiazepine antagonist; reverses sedative effects of benzodiazepines used in conscious sedation and general anesthesia; treatment of benzodiazepine overdose

Emergency Dosage Adults: I.V.: Management of benzodiazepine overdose: 0.2 mg initially, followed by 0.1 mg per minute, up to a total of 1 mg

Note: Avoid use in patients who receive benzodiazepines on a chronic basis; duration of flumazenil's effect (-1 hour) is often shorter than that of most benzodiazepines, and patient should be monitored for resedation; it should also be noted that respiratory depression may not be improved, however mental status should improve

Usual Dosage Resedation: Repeated doses may be given at 20-minute intervals as needed; repeat treatment doses of 1 mg (at a rate of 0.5 mg/minute) should be given at any time and no more than 3 mg should be given in any hour. After intoxication with high doses of benzodiazepines, the duration of a single dose of flumazenil is not expected to exceed 1 hour; if desired, the period of wakefulness may be prolonged with repeated low intravenous doses of flumazenil, or by an infusion of 0.1-0.4 mg/hour. Most patients with benzodiazepine overdose will respond to a cumulative dose of 1-3 mg and doses >3 mg do not reliably produce additional effects. Rarely, patients with a partial response at 3 mg may require additional titration up to a total dose of 5 mg. **If a patient has not responded 5 minutes after receiving a cumulative dose of 5 mg, the major cause of sedation is not likely to be due to benzodiazepines.**

Mechanism of Action Antagonizes the effect of benzodiazepines on the GABA/benzodiazepine receptor complex. Flumazenil is benzodiazepine specific and does not antagonize other nonbenzodiazepine GABA agonists (including ethanol, barbiturates, general anesthetics); flumazenil does not reverse the effects of opiates

GELATIN (Absorbable)

Therapeutic Category Hemostatic Agent
Use Adjunct to provide hemostasis in surgery; open prostatic surgery
Usual Dosage Hemostasis: Apply packs or sponges dry or saturated with sodium chloride. When applied dry, hold in place with moderate pressure. When applied wet, squeeze to remove air bubbles. The powder is applied as a paste prepared by adding approximately 4 mL of sterile saline solution to the powder.

GLUCAGON

Therapeutic Category Antidote; Diagnostic Agent
Use Management of hypoglycemia; diagnostic aid in radiologic examinations to temporarily inhibit GI tract movement
Usual Dosage

Hypoglycemia or insulin shock therapy: I.M., I.V., SubQ:
Children <20 kg: 0.5 mg or 20-30 mcg/kg/dose; repeated in 20 minutes as needed
Children ≥20 kg and Adults: 1 mg; may repeat in 20 minutes as needed

Note: I.V. dextrose should be administered as soon as it is available; if patient fails to respond to glucagon, I.V. dextrose must be given.

Beta-blocker overdose, calcium channel blocker overdose (unlabeled use): Adults: I.V.: 5-10 mg over 1 minutes followed by an infusion of 1-10 mg/hour. The following has also been reported for beta-blocker overdose: 3-10 mg or initially 0.5-5 mg bolus followed by continuous infusion 1-5 mg/hour

Diagnostic aid: Adults: I.M., I.V.: 0.25-2 mg 10 minutes prior to procedure

Mechanism of Action Stimulates adenylate cyclase to produce increased cyclic AMP, which promotes hepatic glycogenolysis and gluconeogenesis, causing a raise in blood glucose levels

GLUCOSE

Therapeutic Category Antihypoglycemic Agent
Use Management of hypoglycemia
Usual Dosage Adults: Oral: 10-20 g

HYDROCORTISONE

Therapeutic Category Anti-inflammatory Agent; Corticosteroid, Systemic; Corticosteroid, Topical (Low Potency)

Use

Dental: Treatment of a variety of oral diseases of allergic, inflammatory or autoimmune origin

Medical: Management of adrenocortical insufficiency

Emergency Dosage Moderate to severe anaphylaxis, to prevent late-phase recurrence of symptoms: I.V. push: 100 mg

Usual Dosage Adults: Anti-inflammatory or immunosuppressive: Adolescents and Adults: Oral, I.M., I.V.: Succinate: 15-240 mg every 12 hours

Mechanism of Action Decreases inflammation by suppression of migration of polymorphonuclear leukocytes and reversal of increased capillary permeability

LORAZEPAM

Therapeutic Category Benzodiazepine

Use

Oral: Management of anxiety disorders or short-term (≤4 months) relief of the symptoms of anxiety or anxiety associated with depressive symptoms

I.V.: Status epilepticus, preanesthesia for desired amnesia

Usual Dosage

Antiemetic (unlabeled use):

Children 2-15 years: I.V.: 0.05 mg/kg (up to 2 mg/dose) prior to chemotherapy

Adults: Oral, I.V. (**Note**: May be administered sublingually; not a labeled route): 0.5-2 mg every 4-6 hours as needed

Anxiety and sedation (unlabeled in children except for oral use in children >12 years):

Infants and Children: Oral, I.M., I.V.: Usual: 0.05 mg/kg/dose (range: 0.02-0.09 mg/kg) every 4-8 hours

I.V.: May use smaller doses (eg, 0.01-0.03 mg/kg) and repeat every 20 minutes, as needed to titrate to effect

Adults: Oral: 1-10 mg/day in 2-3 divided doses; usual dose: 2-6 mg/day in divided doses

Elderly: 0.5-4 mg/day; initial dose not to exceed 2 mg

Insomnia: Adults: Oral: 2-4 mg at bedtime

Preoperative: Adults:

I.M.: 0.05 mg/kg administered 2 hours before surgery (maximum: 4 mg/dose)

I.V.: 0.044 mg/kg 15-20 minutes before surgery (usual maximum: 2 mg/dose)

Preprocedural anxiety (dental use): Adults: Oral: 1-2 mg 1 hour before procedure

Operative amnesia: Adults: I.V.: Up to 0.05 mg/kg (maximum: 4 mg/dose)

Sedation (preprocedure): Infants and Children (unlabeled):

Oral, I.M., I.V.: Usual: 0.05 mg/kg (range: 0.02-0.09 mg/kg)

I.V.: May use smaller doses (eg, 0.01-0.03 mg/kg) and repeat every 20 minutes, as needed to titrate to effect

Status epilepticus: I.V.:

Infants and Children (unlabeled): 0.1 mg/kg slow I.V. over 2-5 minutes; do not exceed 4 mg/single dose; may repeat second dose of 0.05 mg/kg slow I.V. in 10-15 minutes if needed

Adolescents: 0.07 mg/kg slow I.V. over 2-5 minutes; maximum: 4 mg/dose; may repeat in 10-15 minutes

Adults: 4 mg/dose slow I.V. over 2-5 minutes; may repeat in 10-15 minutes; usual maximum dose: 8 mg

Rapid tranquilization of agitated patient (administer every 30-60 minutes): Adults:

Oral: 1-2 mg

I.M.: 0.5-1 mg

Average total dose for tranquilization: Oral, I.M.: 4-8 mg

Agitation in the ICU patient (unlabeled): Adults:

I.V.: 0.02-0.06 mg/kg every 2-6 hours

I.V. infusion: 0.01-0.1 mg/kg/hour

Dosage adjustment in renal impairment: I.V.: Risk of propylene glycol toxicity. Monitor closely if using for prolonged periods of time or at high doses.

Dosage adjustment in hepatic impairment: Use cautiously.

Mechanism of Action Binds to stereospecific benzodiazepine receptors on the postsynaptic GABA neuron at several sites within the central nervous system, including the limbic system, reticular formation. Enhancement of the inhibitory effect of GABA on neuronal excitability results by increased neuronal membrane permeability to chloride ions. This shift in chloride ions results in hyperpolarization (a less excitable state) and stabilization.

METHYLPREDNISOLONE

Therapeutic Category Corticosteroid, Systemic

Use Treatment of a variety of oral diseases of allergic, inflammatory, or autoimmune origin

Usual Dosage Dosing should be based on the lesser of ideal body weight or actual body weight

Only sodium succinate may be given I.V.; methylprednisolone sodium succinate is highly soluble and has a rapid effect by I.M. and I.V. routes. Methylprednisolone acetate has a low solubility and has a sustained I.M. effect.

Children:

Anti-inflammatory or immunosuppressive: Oral, I.M., I.V. (sodium succinate): 0.5-1.7 mg/kg/day or 5-25 mg/m^2/day in divided doses every 6-12 hours; "Pulse" therapy: 15-30 mg/kg/dose over ≥30 minutes given once daily for 3 days

Asthma exacerbations, including status asthmaticus (emergency medical care or hospital doses) (NIH Asthma Guidelines, NAEPP, 2007): Children ≤12 years: Oral, I.V.: 1-2 mg/kg/day in 2 divided doses (maximum: 60 mg/day) until peak expiratory flow is 70% of predicted or personal best

Lupus nephritis: I.V. (sodium succinate): 30 mg/kg over ≥30 minutes every other day for 6 doses

Adults:

Anti-inflammatory or immunosuppressive:

Oral: 2-60 mg/day in 1-4 divided doses to start, followed by gradual reduction in dosage to the lowest possible level consistent with maintaining an adequate clinical response.

I.M. (sodium succinate): 10-80 mg/day once daily

I.M. (acetate): 10-80 mg every 1-2 weeks

I.V. (sodium succinate): 10-40 mg over a period of several minutes and repeated I.V. or I.M. at intervals depending on clinical response; when high dosages are needed, give 30 mg/kg over a period ≥30 minutes and may be repeated every 4-6 hours for 48 hours.

Asthma exacerbations, including status asthmaticus (emergency medical care or hospital doses): Oral, I.V.: 40-80 mg/day in 1-2 divided doses until peak expiratory flow is 70% of predicted or personal best (NIH Asthma Guidelines, NAEPP, 2007)

Lupus nephritis: High-dose "pulse" therapy: I.V. (sodium succinate): 1 g/day for 3 days

Pneumocystis pneumonia in AIDs patients: I.V.: 40-60 mg every 6 hours for 7-10 days

Mechanism of Action In a tissue-specific manner, corticosteroids regulate gene expression subsequent to binding specific intracellular receptors and translocation into the nucleus. Corticosteroids exert a wide array of physiologic effects including modulation of carbohydrate, protein, and lipid metabolism and maintenance of fluid and electrolyte homeostasis. Moreover cardiovascular, immunologic, musculoskeletal, endocrine, and neurologic physiology are influenced by corticosteroids. Decreases inflammation by suppression of migration of polymorphonuclear leukocytes and reversal of increased capillary permeability.

MICROFIBRILLAR COLLAGEN HEMOSTAT

Therapeutic Category Hemostatic Agent

Use Adjunct to hemostasis when control of bleeding by ligature is ineffective or impractical

Usual Dosage Apply dry directly to source of bleeding; remove excess material after 10-15 minutes

Mechanism of Action Collagen hemostat is an absorbable topical hemostatic agent prepared from purified bovine corium collagen and shredded into fibrils. Physically, microfibrillar collagen hemostat yields a large surface area. Chemically, it is collagen with hydrochloric acid noncovalently bound to some of the available amino groups in the collagen molecules. When in contact with a bleeding surface, collagen hemostat attracts platelets which adhere to its fibrils and undergo the release phenomenon. This triggers aggregation of the platelets into thrombi in the interstices of the fibrous mass, initiating the formation of a physiologic platelet plug.

MORPHINE SULFATE

Therapeutic Category Analgesic, Opioid

Use Relief of moderate to severe acute and chronic pain; pain of myocardial infarction; relieves dyspnea of acute left ventricular failure and pulmonary edema; preanesthetic medication

Emergency Dosage Acute myocardial infarction: I.V., S.L.: 2-4 mg

Usual Dosage These are guidelines and do not represent the doses that may be required in all patients. Doses and dosage intervals should be titrated to pain relief/prevention.

Children >6 months and <50 kg: Acute pain (moderate-to-severe):

Oral (immediate release formulations): 0.15-0.3 mg/kg every 3-4 hours as needed. Note: The American Pain Society recommends an initial dose of 0.3 mg/kg for children with severe pain.

I.M., I.V.: 0.1-0.2 mg/kg every 3-4 hours as needed

I.V. infusion: Range: 10-60 mcg/kg/hour

Patient-controlled analgesia (PCA) (American Pain Society, 2008): Note: Opiate-naive: Consider lower end of dosing range:

Usual concentration: 1 mg/mL

Demand dose: Usual: 0.02 mg/kg/dose; range: 0.01-0.03 mg/kg/dose

Lockout interval: 6-8 minutes

Usual basal rate: 0-0.03 mg/kg/hour

Adults:

Oral (immediate release formulations): Opiate-naive: Initial: 10 mg every 4 hours as needed; patients with prior opiate exposure may require higher initial doses: usual dosage range: 10-30 mg every 4 hours as needed

I.M., SubQ: Note: Repeated SubQ administration causes local tissue irritation, pain, and induration.

Initial: Opiate-naive: 5-10 mg every 4 hours as needed; patients with prior opiate exposure may require higher initial doses; usual dosage range: 5-20 mg every 4 hours as needed

Epidural: Initial: 5 mg in lumbar region; if inadequate pain relief within 1 hour, give 1-2 mg, maximum dose: 10 mg/24 hours

Intrathecal (1/10 of epidural dose): 0.2-1 mg/dose; repeat doses not recommended

Rectal: 10-20 mg every 4 hours

Mechanism of Action Binds to opiate receptors in the CNS, causing inhibition of ascending pain pathways, altering the perception of and response to pain; produces generalized CNS depression

NALOXONE

Therapeutic Category Antidote; Opioid Antagonist

Use

Dental: Reverses CNS and respiratory depressant effects of fentanyl and meperidine during I.V. conscious state

Medical: Reverses CNS and respiratory depression in suspected narcotic overdose; neonatal opiate depression; coma of unknown etiology

Emergency Dosage I.V.: 0.4-2 mg; may be repeated at 2- to 3-minute intervals up to 10 mg; I.M. or SubQ administration may be used if I.V. administration is not possible, but response may be delayed

Usual Dosage Adults: Narcotic overdose: I.V.: 0.4-2 mg every 2-3 minutes as needed; may need to repeat doses every 20-60 minutes, if no response is observed after 10 mg, question the diagnosis. **Note**: Use 0.1-0.2 mg increments in patients who are opioid-dependent and in postoperative patients to avoid large cardiovascular changes.

Mechanism of Action Pure opioid antagonist that competes and displaces narcotics at opioid receptor sites

NITROGLYCERIN

Therapeutic Category Vasodilator

Use Treatment of angina pectoris; I.V. for congestive heart failure (especially when associated with acute myocardial infarction); pulmonary hypertension; hypertensive emergencies occurring perioperatively (especially during cardiovascular surgery)

Emergency Dosage Angina pectoris or acute myocardial infarction: Sublingual: 0.2-0.6 mg, may be repeated in 5 minutes, up to 3 times over 15 minutes

Usual Dosage Note: Hemodynamic and antianginal tolerance often develop within 24-48 hours of continuous nitrate administration

Children: Pulmonary hypertension: Continuous infusion: Start 0.25-0.5 mcg/kg/minute and titrate by 1 mcg/kg/minute at 20- to 60-minute intervals to desired effect; usual dose: 1-3 mcg/kg/minute; maximum: 5 mcg/kg/minute

Adults:

Oral: 2.5-9 mg 2-4 times/day (up to 26 mg 4 times/day)

I.V.: 5 mcg/minute, increase by 5 mcg/minute every 3-5 minutes to 20 mcg/minute; if no response at 20 mcg/minute increase by 10 mcg/minute every 3-5 minutes, up to 200 mcg/minute

Ointment: 1" to 2" every 8 hours up to 4" to 5" every 4 hours

Patch, transdermal: 0.2-0.4 mg/hour initially and titrate to doses of 0.4-0.8 mg/hour; tolerance is minimized by using a patch-on period of 12-14 hours and patch-off period of 10-12 hours

Sublingual: 0.2-0.6 mg every 5 minutes for maximum of 3 doses in 15 minutes; may also use prophylactically 5-10 minutes prior to activities which may provoke an attack

Translingual: 1-2 sprays into mouth under tongue every 3-5 minutes for maximum of 3 doses in 15 minutes; may also be used 5-10 minutes prior to activities which may provoke an attack prophylactically

May need to use nitrate-free interval (10-12 hours/day) to avoid tolerance development; tolerance may possibly be reversed with acetylcysteine; gradually decrease dose in patients receiving NTG for prolonged period to avoid withdrawal reaction

Mechanism of Action Reduces cardiac oxygen demand by decreasing left ventricular pressure and systemic vascular resistance; dilates coronary arteries and improves collateral flow to ischemic regions

OXYGEN

Therapeutic Category Dental Gases

Use

Dental: Administered as a supplement with nitrous oxide to ensure adequate ventilation during sedation; a resuscitative agent for medical emergencies in dental office

Medical: Treatment of various clinical disorders, both respiratory and nonrespiratory; relief of arterial hypoxia and secondary complications; treatment of pulmonary hypertension, polycythemia secondary to hypoxemia, chronic disease states complicated by anemia, cancer, migraine headaches, coronary artery disease, seizure disorders, sickle-cell crisis and sleep apnea.

Usual Dosage Children and Adults: Average rate of 2 L/minute

Mechanism of Action Increased oxygen in tidal volume and oxygenation of tissues at molecular level

PROMETHAZINE

Therapeutic Category Antiemetic; Histamine H_1 Antagonist; Histamine H_1 Antagonist, First Generation

Use Symptomatic treatment of various allergic conditions; antiemetic; motion sickness; sedative; adjunct to postoperative analgesia and anesthesia

Usual Dosage

Children ≥2 years:

Allergic conditions: Oral, rectal: 0.1 mg/kg/dose (maximum: 12.5 mg) every 6 hours during the day and 0.5 mg/kg/dose (maximum: 25 mg) at bedtime as needed

Antiemetic: Oral, I.M., I.V., rectal: 0.25-1 mg/kg 4-6 times/day as needed (maximum: 25 mg/dose)

Motion sickness: Oral, rectal: 0.5 mg/kg/dose 30 minutes to 1 hour before departure, then every 12 hours as needed (maximum dose: 25 mg twice daily)

Preoperative analgesia/hypnotic adjunct: I.M., I.V.: 1.1 mg/kg in combination with an analgesic or hypnotic (at reduced doses) and an atropine-like agent. Note: Dose should not exceed half of suggested adult dose

Sedation: Oral, I.M., I.V., rectal: 0.5-1 mg/kg/dose every 6 hours as needed (maximum: 50 mg/dose)

Adults:

Allergic conditions (including allergic reactions to blood or plasma):

Oral, rectal: 25 mg at bedtime or 12.5 mg before meals and at bedtime (range: 6.25-12.5 mg 3 times/day)

I.M., I.V.: 25 mg, may repeat in 2 hours when necessary; switch to oral route as soon as feasible

Antiemetic: Oral, I.M., I.V., rectal: 12.5-25 mg every 4-6 hours as needed

Motion sickness: Oral, rectal: 25 mg 30-60 minutes before departure, then every 12 hours as needed

Pre-/postoperative analgesia/hypnotic adjunct: I.M., I.V.: 25-50 mg in combination with analgesic or hypnotic (at reduced dosage)

Sedation: Oral, I.M., I.V., rectal: 12.5-50 mg/dose

Mechanism of Action Blocks postsynaptic mesolimbic dopaminergic receptors in the brain; exhibits a strong alpha-adrenergic blocking effect and depresses the release of hypothalamic and hypophyseal hormones; competes with histamine for the H1-receptor; reduces stimuli to the brainstem reticular system

THROMBIN (Topical)

Therapeutic Category Hemostatic Agent

Use Hemostasis whenever minor bleeding from capillaries and small venules is accessible

Usual Dosage Topical: Hemostasis: Note: For topical use only; do not administer intravenously or intra-arterially:

Evithrom™: Children and Adults: Dose depends on area to be treated; up to 10 mL was used with absorbable gelatin sponge in clinical studies

Recothrom™: Adults: Dose depends on area to be treated

Thrombi-Gel® 10, 40, 100: Adults: Wet product with up to 3 mL, 10 mL, or 20 mL, respectively, of 0.9% sodium chloride or SWFI; apply directly over source of the bleeding with manual pressure

Thrombi-Pad®: Adults: Apply pad directly over source of bleeding; may apply dry or wetted with up to 10 mL of 0.9% sodium chloride. If desired, product may be left in place for up to 24 hours; do not leave in the body.

Thrombin-JMI®: Adults:

Solution: Use 1000-2000 int. units/mL of solution where bleeding is profuse; use 100 int. units/mL for bleeding from skin or mucosal surfaces

Powder: May apply powder directly to the site of bleeding or on oozing surfaces

Mechanism of Action Activates platelets and catalyzes the conversion of fibrinogen to fibrin to promote hemostasis

TRANEXAMIC ACID

Therapeutic Category Antifibrinolytic Agent; Antihemophilic Agent; Hemostatic Agent; Lysine Analog

Use

Solution for injection: Short-term use (2-8 days) in hemophilia patients to reduce or prevent hemorrhage and reduce need for replacement therapy during and following tooth extraction

Tablet: Treatment of cyclic heavy menstrual bleeding

Usual Dosage

I.V.:

Children and Adults: Tooth extraction in patients with hemophilia (in combination with replacement therapy): 10 mg/kg immediately before surgery, then 10 mg/kg/dose 3-4 times/day; may be used for 2-8 days

Adults: Trauma-associated hemorrhage (unlabeled use): Loading dose: 1000 mg over 10 minutes, followed by 1000 mg over the next 8 hours. Note: Clinical trial included patients with significant hemorrhage (SBP <90 mm Hg, heart rate >110 bpm, or both) or those at risk of significant hemorrhage. Treatment began within 8 hours of injury (CRASH-2 Trial Collaborators, 2010).

Oral: Adults: Menorrhagia: 1300 mg 3 times daily (3900 mg/day) for up to 5 days during monthly menstruation

Mechanism of Action Forms a reversible complex that displaces plasminogen from fibrin resulting in inhibition of fibrinolysis; it also inhibits the proteolytic activity of plasmin

SECTION TWO: DENTAL OFFICE MEDICAL EMERGENCIES

ALL PRACTITIONERS MUST BE PREPARED TO CARRY OUT A BASIC PLAN FOR STABILIZATION

> THESE STEPS ARE THE BASIC ACTION PLAN FOR STABILIZATION IN EVERY OFFICE EMERGENCY. THESE STEPS SHOULD BE ACTIVATED WITHIN THE FIRST SECONDS FOLLOWING RECOGNITION OF ANY DEVELOPING PROBLEM SOMETIMES BASED ON THE INITIAL RECOGNITION SIGNS, ACTIVATION OF THE EMERGENCY MEDICAL SYSTEM WOULD OCCUR IMMEDIATELY - USUALLY BY CALLING 911 (IF AVAILABLE IN YOUR AREA).

> IF THE DENTIST IS UNSURE OF THE UNDERLYING REASON FOR THE MEDICAL EMERGENCY OR DOES NOT FEEL ADEQUATELY TRAINED, THEN BASIC LIFE SUPPORT (BLS) PROCEDURES SHOULD BE THE EXTENT OF THE TREATMENT UNTIL THE EMERGENCY MEDICAL TEAM ARRIVES.

BASIC ACTION PLAN FOR STABILIZATION

PATIENT PLACEMENT →

- UPRIGHT / SEMI-RECLINING?
- SUPINE?
- TRENDELENBURG (FEET UP, HEAD DOWN)*?

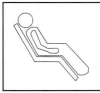
Upright / Semireclining

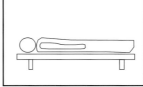
Supine

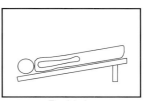
Trendelenburg

AIRWAY AND BREATHING →

- IS THE AIRWAY OPEN?
- CLEAR OF OBSTRUCTIONS?
- IS THE PATIENT BREATHING ON HIS/HER OWN?
- DOES THE SITUATION REQUIRE OXYGEN TO INCREASE PERFUSION?
- ACTIVATE EMS IF NECESSARY

CIRCULATION →

- MONITOR PULSE, MEASURE BLOOD PRESSURE
- PROCEED WITH BLS, IF APPROPRIATE (see pages 13-15)

ADDITIONAL MANAGEMENT† →

- ALWAYS CONSIDER ACTIVATING EMS IMMEDIATELY
- CONTINUALLY OBSERVE, MONITOR VITAL SIGNS, AND EVALUATE FOR ANY SIGNS OF RECOVERY OR DETERIORATION
- ASSIGN SOMEONE IN THE OFFICE TO QUICKLY RE-EVALUATE PATIENT'S HISTORY AND RECORD FOR CLUES TO THE CAUSE OF THE INCIDENT OR DRUGS THE PATIENT MAY BE TAKING
- DETERMINE, IF POSSIBLE, THE TENTATIVE MEDICAL CONDITION CAUSING THE SYMPTOMS
- DELIVER SPECIFIC CARE, IF APPROPRIATE
- BE PREPARED TO ACTIVATE EMS (CALL FOR ASSISTANCE) IF PATIENT'S CONDITION DETERIORATES
- ALWAYS CONSIDER THE NEED FOR FOLLOW-UP MEDICAL EVALUATION AS PATIENT RECOVERS

*Trendelenburg's position is a supine position which is inclined at an angle so that the pelvis and legs are slightly higher than the head.
†Although these management suggestions are essentially the same for each of the protocols, the order and specific care will vary.

LOSS OF CONSCIOUSNESS

MOST COMMON

Syncope (Vasovagal Syncope or Simple Fainting)

Postural (Orthostatic) Hypotension

Hypoglycemia (Insulin Shock)

OTHER EMERGENCIES WHICH MAY INVOLVE LOSS OF CONSCIOUSNESS

Anaphylactic Shock

Stroke / Cerebrovascular Accident

Seizure Disorders

SYNCOPE (Vasovagal Syncope or Simple Fainting)

Cause: Decreased circulation of blood to the brain
(may be associated with events such as emotional upset, anxiety, starting an I.V., blood draw)

SYMPTOMS: Anxiety, pallor, diaphoresis (cold and clammy), rapid pulse (tachycardia) followed by bradycardia, decreased blood pressure (transient increase in blood pressure followed by rapid decrease), loss of consciousness, dilatation of pupils, nausea

TREATMENT:

PATIENT PLACEMENT	→	**TRENDELENBURG (FEET UP, HEAD DOWN)**
AIRWAY AND BREATHING	→	**MAINTAIN OPEN AIRWAY**
	→	**ADMINISTERING OXYGEN MAY ASSIST IN RECOVERY**
CIRCULATION	→	**MONITOR PULSE**
ADDITIONAL MANAGEMENT	→	**IF UNSURE THAT SYMPTOMS ARE CONSISTENT WITH SYNCOPE, CONSIDER ACTIVATING EMS IMMEDIATELY**
	→	**PLACE CRUSHED AMMONIA CAPSULE UNDER NOSE**
	→	**APPLY COLD COMPRESS TO FOREHEAD OR TO BACK OF NECK**
	→	**MONITOR VITAL SIGNS**
	→	**ACTIVATE EMS CALL FOR ASSISTANCE IF PATIENT'S CONDITION IS UNSTABLE OR IF THERE IS A DELAY IN RESPONSE**
	→	**REASSURE AND COMFORT PATIENT WHEN THEY AWAKEN, COVER WITH BLANKET FOR WARMTH**
	→	**CHECK PATIENT'S RECORD FOR MEDICATIONS WITH A PREDISPOSITION TO SYNCOPE**

SIGNS WHEN PATIENT IS RECOVERING

- Patient awakens; vital signs remain stable

SIGNS WHEN PATIENT IS DETERIORATING

- Patient does not awaken after ~1 minute; vital signs are unstable; re-evaluate diagnosis (consider hypoglycemia, seizure, cardiac arrest, anaphylaxis, or cerebrovascular accident (CVA), transient ischemic attack (TIA)

NOTE: Patient may require referral for syncope workup if problem is recurrent or if the cause is unclear.

MEDICATIONS WITH ELEVATED INCIDENCE OF SYNCOPE*
AS AN ADVERSE REACTION

Generic Name	U.S. Brand Name	Canadian Brand Name
SYNCOPE >10%		
Doxazosin mesylate	Cardura® Tablets (0.5% to 23%)	
Fluorescein sodium	AK-Fluor® Injection (10% and 25%)	
Terazosin hydrochloride	Hytrin® (0.5% to 21%)	
SYNCOPE 1% to 10%		
Aldesleukin	Proleukin® Injection (3%)	
Alprazolam	Xanax® Tablets (3.1% to 3.8%)	Nu-Alprax
Amlodipine besylate	Norvasc® Tablets (>0.1% to 1%)	
Amphotericin B cholesteryl sulfate complex	Amphotec® Injection (1% to 5%)	
Anagrelide hydrochloride	Agrylin® Capsules (1% to 5%)	
Atorvastatin	Lipitor® Tablets (<2 %)	
Betaxolol	Kerlone® Tablets (<2%)	
Brimonidine tartrate	Alphagan® Ophthalmic Solution (<3%)	
Budesonide	Pulmicort Turbuhaler® Inhalation Powder (1% to 3%)	Entocort®
Cabergoline	Dostinex® Tablets (1% to <10%)	
Carvedilol	Coreg® Tablets (3.4%)	
Clomipramine hydrochloride	Anafranil® Capsules (≤2%)	Apo®-Clomipramine
Clozapine	Clozaril® Tablets (>5% to 6%)	
Daunorubicin citrate liposome	DaunoXome® (≤5%)	
Delavirdine mesylate	Rescriptor® Tablets (<2%)	
Disopyramide phosphate	Norpace® (1% to 3%)	
Donepezil hydrochloride	Aricept® Tablets (2%)	
Estradiol	Estring® Vaginal Ring (1% to 3%)	
Flecainide acetate	Tambocor™ Tablets (1% to 3%)	
Flunisolide	Aerobid®/Aerobid®-M Inhaler Systems (1% to 3%)	Bronalid®
Glipizide	Glucotrol® XL Extended Release Tablets (<3%)	
Guanadrel sulfate	Hylorel® Tablets (7.8%)	
Immune globulin, intravenous	Gamimune® N 5%, Solvent/ Detergent-Treated	
Immune globulin, intravenous	Gamimune® N 10%, Solvent/ Detergent-Treated	
Interferon alfa-2a, recombinant	Roferon-A® Injection (<0.5% to 5%)	
Interferon alfa-2b	Intron® A Injection (<5%)	
Interferon beta-1a	Avonex™ (4%)	
Leuprolide acetate	Lupron Depot-3® Month (<5%)	
Leuprolide acetate	Lupron Depot-Ped™ (<2%)	
Leuprolide acetate	Lupron® Injection (<5%)	
Leuprolide acetate	Lupron® Injection Pediatric (<2%)	
Misoprostol	Crixivan® Capsules (<2%)	
Moricizine hydrochloride	Ethmozine® Tablets (<2%)	
Morphine sulfate, sustained release	Kadian™ Capsules (<3%)	Epimorph®
Nilutamide	Nilandron™ Tablets (2%)	Anandron®
Nitroglycerin	Transderm-Nitro® Transdermal Therapeutic System (4%)	
Pamidronate disodium	Aredia® Injection (≤6%)	
Pentostatin	Nipent™ Injection (<3%)	
Pergolide mesylate	Permax® Tablets (2.1%)	
Prazosin hydrochloride	Minipress® Capsules (1% to 4%)	Novo-Prazin
Progesterone	Crinone™ (<5%)	PMS-Progesterone®
Propafenone hydrochloride	Rythmol® Tablets (2.2%)	
Ritonavir	Norvir® Capsules, Oral Solution (<2%)	
Saquinavir mesylate	Invirase® Capsules (<2%)	
Sotalol	Betapace® Tablets (1% to 5%)	Sotacor®
Trazodone hydrochloride	Desyrel® (2.8% to 4.5%)	
Verapamil hydrochloride, extended release	Covera®-HS Tablets (<2%)	Nu-Verap

*From manufacturer's professional package insert; drugs causing postural or orthostatic hypotension are included in a separate table. For the sake of brevity, this list has been limited to medications with an incidence of >1%. Many other medications in similar therapeutic categories cite such reactions as <1%.

POSTURAL (ORTHOSTATIC) HYPOTENSION

Cause: *Rapid fall in blood pressure when moving from the supine to upright position*

SYMPTOMS: Similar to simple fainting, however related to positioning

TREATMENT:

PATIENT PLACEMENT	→	**IMMEDIATELY RETURN PATIENT TO SUPINE POSITION, OR TRENDELENBURG IF POSSIBLE**
AIRWAY AND BREATHING	→	**MAINTAIN OPEN AIRWAY**
	→	**ADMINISTERING OXYGEN MAY ASSIST IN RECOVERY**
CIRCULATION	→	**MONITOR PULSE**
ADDITIONAL MANAGEMENT	→	**IF UNSURE, CONSIDER ACTIVATING EMS IMMEDIATELY**
	→	**MONITOR VITAL SIGNS**
	→	**IF PATIENT HAS NOT RESPONDED TO REPOSITIONING, MANAGE AS SIMPLE FAINTING WITH AMMONIA CAPSULE AND COLD COMPRESS**
	→	**REPOSITION PATIENT SLOWLY AFTER STABLE**
	→	**ACTIVATE EMS - CALL FOR ASSISTANCE IF PATIENT'S CONDITION DETERIORATES**
	→	**CHECK PATIENT'S RECORD FOR MEDICATIONS WITH A PREDISPOSITION TO POSTURAL (ORTHOSTATIC) HYPOTENSION** (see reverse of this page)

SIGNS WHEN PATIENT IS RECOVERING

- Patient awakens or becomes more alert; vital signs remain stable

SIGNS WHEN PATIENT IS DETERIORATING

- Patient completely loses consciousness; vital signs are unstable; re-evaluate diagnosis – consider hypoglycemia, seizure, cardiac arrest, anaphylaxis, or cerebrovascular accident (CVA), transient ischemic attack (TIA)

MEDICATIONS WITH ELEVATED INCIDENCE OF POSTURAL OR ORTHOSTATIC HYPOTENSION* AS AN ADVERSE REACTION

Generic Name	U.S. Brand Name	Canadian Brand Name
HYPOTENSION, ORTHOSTATIC >10%		
Clomipramine hydrochloride	Anafranil® Capsules (~20%)	Apo®-Clomipramine
Doxazosin mesylate	Cardura® Tablets (≤23%)	
HYPOTENSION, ORTHOSTATIC 1% to 10%		
Amantadine hydrochloride	Symmetrel® Capsules, Syrup (1% to 5%)	Endantadine®
Bromocriptine mesylate	Parlodel® (6%)	Apo®-Bromocriptine
Cabergoline	Dostinex® Tablets (4%)	
Carbidopa / levodopa	Sinemet® CR Tablets (1%)	
Enalapril maleate	Vasotec® Tablets (0.5% to 1.6%)	Apo®-Enalapril
Enalapril maleate / hydrochlorothiazide	Vaseretic® Tablets (0.5% to 2%)	
Fosinopril	Monopril® Tablets (1.4% to 1.9%)	
Guanadrel sulfate	Hylorel® Tablets (6.6% to 7.5%)	
Itraconazole	Sporanox® Capsules (1%)	
Ivermectin	Stromectol® Tablets (1.1%)	
Lisinopril	Zestril® Tablets (0.3% to 1.2%)	Apo®-Lisinopril
Lisinopril / hydrochlorothiazide	Zestoretic® Tablets (0.3% to 1%)	
Metolazone	Mykrox® Tablets (<2%)	
Nifedipine	Adalat® Capsules (~5%)	Adalat PA®
Prazosin	Minipress® Capsules (1% to 4%)	Novo-Prazin
Ritonavir	Norvir® Capsules, Oral Solution (<2%)	
HYPOTENSION, POSTURAL >10%		
Clonidine hydrochloride	Duraclon® Injection (31.6% to 47%)	ixarit®
Doxazosin mesylate	Cardura® Tablets (0.3% to ≤29%)	
Labetalol hydrochloride	Normodyne® Injection (58%)	
Labetalol hydrochloride	Trandate® Injection (58%)	
Tacrolimus	Prograf® Capsules (3% to 15%)	
Terazosin hydrochloride	Hytrin® Capsules (0.5% to 21%)	
HYPOTENSION, POSTURAL 1% to 10%		
Amphotericin B cholesteryl sulfate complex	Amphotec® Injection (≥5%)	
Anagrelide hydrochloride	Agrylin® Capsules (1% to 5%)	
Atenolol	Tenormin® Tablets, Injection (2% to 4%)	Taro-Atenol®
Atenolol / chlorthalidone	Tenoretic® Tablets (2% to 4%)	
Atorvastatin	Lipitor® Tablets (<2%)	
Bromocriptine mesylate	Parlodel® Tablets (6%)	Apo®-Bromocriptine
Carvedilol	Coreg® Tablets (<1% to 9.7%)	
Clomipramine hydrochloride	Anafranil® Capsules (4% to 6%)	Apo®-Clomipramine
Divalproex sodium, delayed release	Depakote® Tablets (1% to 5%)	Deproic
Enalaprilat	Vasotec® I.V. (2.3%)	
Ibutilide fumarate	Corvert® Injection (2%)	
Labetalol hydrochloride	Trandate® Tablets (1%)	
Morphine sulfate, sustained release	Kadian™ Tablets (<3%)	Epimorph®
Mycophenolate mofetil	CellCept® Capsules (3%)	
Nefazodone hydrochloride	Serzone® Tablets (2.8% to 4%)	
Nicardipine hydrochloride	Cardene® I.V. (1.4%)	Ridene
Olanzapine	Zyprexa™ Tablets (5%)	
Oxycodone hydrochloride, controlled release	OxyContin® Tablets (1% to 5%)	Supeudol®
Paroxetine hydrochloride	Paxil™ Tablets (1.2%)	
Pergolide mesylate	Permax® Tablets (9%)	
Ramipril	Altace™ (2.2%)	
Tacrolimus	Prograf® Capsules (3% to 15%)	
Valproate sodium	Depacon® Injection (≥1%)	Deproic
Venlafaxine hydrochloride	Effexor® Tablets (1%)	

*From manufacturer's professional package insert; some use "postural" and others use "orthostatic" to identify this form of hypotension.

For the sake of brevity, this list has been limited to medications with an incidence of >1%. Many other medications in similar therapeutic categories cite such reactions as <1%.

HYPOGLYCEMIA (INSULIN SHOCK)

Cause: Acute hypoglycemia associated with oral hypoglycemics or excess insulin

SYMPTOMS: Sudden onset, confusion, nervousness, diaphoresis (cold and clammy), drooling from mouth, full and bounding pulse, convulsions (not common), pallor, loss of consciousness/coma

TREATMENT:

PATIENT PLACEMENT	→	**SEMI-RECLINING (SUPINE IF PATIENT LOSES CONSCIOUSNESS)**
AIRWAY AND BREATHING	→	**MAINTAIN OPEN AIRWAY**
	→	**ADMINISTERING OXYGEN WILL NOT HURT, BUT USUALLY IS NOT NECESSARY**
CIRCULATION	→	**MONITOR PULSE AND BLOOD PRESSURE**
ADDITIONAL MANAGEMENT	→	**IF UNSURE, CONSIDER ACTIVATING EMS IMMEDIATELY**
	→	**CHECK PATIENT'S RECORD FOR MEDICATIONS**
	→	**MONITOR VITAL SIGNS**
	→	**ADMINISTER ORAL SUGAR (such as orange juice)* NEVER ATTEMPT ORAL ROUTE IF PATIENT IS UNCONSCIOUS (although some practitioners advocate Glutose 15™ oral gel for oral mucosal absorption as long as it does not obstruct airway)**
	→	**IF TRAINED, AND IF PATIENT IS UNCONSCIOUS*, ADMINISTER 50% DEXTROSE I.V., OR CONSIDER I.M. INJECTION OF GLUCAGON IF AVAILABLE**
	→	**ACTIVATE EMS CALL FOR ASSISTANCE IF PATIENT'S CONDITION DETERIORATES**

SIGNS WHEN PATIENT IS RECOVERING

- Patient appears more alert

SIGNS WHEN PATIENT IS DETERIORATING

- Loss of consciousness; vital signs are unstable; re-evaluate diagnosis; consider seizure, cardiac arrest, anaphylaxis, cerebrovascular accident (CVA), or transient ischemic attack (TIA)

*Diabetic acidosis leading to diabetic coma due to prolonged hyperglycemia develops more slowly. Sugar, however, is still the emergency treatment of choice in the unconscious patient until proven otherwise by laboratory evaluation.

SELECTED MEDICATIONS ASSOCIATED WITH HYPOGLYCEMIA

Generic Name	U.S. Brand Name	Canadian Brand Name
Ethanol		
Insulin		

ORAL SULFONYLUREAS AND RELATED HYPOGLYCEMIC AGENTS

Generic Name	U.S. Brand Name	Canadian Brand Name
Acetohexamide	Dymelor®	
Chlorpropamide	Diabenese®	Novo-Propamide
Glimepiride	Amaryl®	
Glipizide	Glucotrol®	
Glyburide	Diaβeta®, Micronase®	Apo®-Glyburide; Euglucon®
Repaglinide	Prandin®	
Tolazamide	Tolinase®	
Tolbutamide	Orinase®	Mobenol®, Novo-Butamide®

OTHER ANTIDIABETIC AGENTS WHICH MAY PROMOTE HYPOGLYCEMIA WHEN USED IN COMBINATION WITH INSULIN AND/OR SULFONYLUREAS

Generic Name	U.S. Brand Name	Canadian Brand Name
Metformin	Glucophage®	Novo-Metformin
Pioglitazone	Actos™	
Rosiglitazone	Avandia®	
Troglitazone	Rezulin®	

Additional notes: Beta-blockers may cause, or worsen, episodes of hypoglycemia and blunt symptoms. A number of medications, including salicylates, co-trimoxazone (high-dose), antidepressants, and antipsychotic agents have been rarely associated with hypoglycemia.

For the sake of brevity, this list has been limited to medications commonly related to incidence of hypoglycemia. Many other medications in similar therapeutic categories cite hypoglycemia as an adverse reaction, although usually at a very low incidence. These reactions are often difficult to attribute to a specific agent.

RESPIRATORY DISTRESS

MOST COMMON

Hyperventilation Syndrome

Asthmatic Attack / Bronchospasm

Airway Obstruction

OTHER EMERGENCIES WHICH MAY INVOLVE LOSS OF CONSCIOUSNESS

Anaphylactic Shock

Acute Myocardial Infarction

Drug Overdoses

HYPERVENTILATION SYNDROME

Cause: *Excessive exhalation of carbon dioxide, producing respiratory alkalosis (can be associated with panic attack/acute anxiety)*

SYMPTOMS: Rapid, shallow breathing, confusion, vertigo (dizziness), paresthesia (numbness or tingling of extremities), carpo-pedal spasm (cramping of hands or feet), chest tightness

TREATMENT:

PATIENT PLACEMENT → **UPRIGHT / SEMI-RECLINING**

AIRWAY AND BREATHING → **MAINTAIN OPEN AIRWAY**

→ **DO NOT ADMINISTER OXYGEN**

CIRCULATION → **MONITOR PULSE AND BLOOD PRESSURE**

ADDITIONAL MANAGEMENT → **IF UNSURE OF HYPERVENTILATION OR IF YOU ARE SUSPICIOUS OF DIABETES (rapid shallow breathing could indicate diabetic acidosis), CONSIDER ACTIVATING EMS IMMEDIATELY**

→ **CALM AND REASSURE THE PATIENT**

→ **INSTRUCT PATIENT TO HOLD BREATH INTO A PAPER BAG TO ENRICH CARBON DIOXIDE, OR TO HOLD BREATH FOR 10 SECONDS THEN BREATHE, THEN REPEAT**

→ **MONITOR VITAL SIGNS**

→ **ACTIVATE EMS - CALL FOR ASSISTANCE IF PATIENT'S CONDITION DETERIORATES**

→ **CHECK PATIENT'S RECORD FOR HISTORY OF PANIC ATTACKS**

SIGNS WHEN PATIENT IS RECOVERING

- Patient's breathing may return to normal

SIGNS WHEN PATIENT IS DETERIORATING

- Patient loses consciousness; vital signs are unstable; re-evaluate diagnosis

ASTHMATIC ATTACK / BRONCHOSPASM

Cause: Spasm and constriction of the bronchi

SYMPTOMS: Labored breathing, wheezing, bronchus spastic cough (coughing spasm), anxiety

TREATMENT:

PATIENT PLACEMENT	→	**UPRIGHT OR AS COMFORTABLE FOR PATIENT**
AIRWAY AND BREATHING	→	**MAINTAIN OPEN AIRWAY**
	→	**BREATHE FOR PATIENT IF NECESSARY**
CIRCULATION	→	**MONITOR PULSE**
ADDITIONAL MANAGEMENT	→	**IF UNSURE, CONSIDER ACTIVATING EMS IMMEDIATELY**
	→	**MONITOR VITAL SIGNS**
	→	**ADMINISTER BRONCHODILATOR (via metered-dose inhaler [MDI]) ALBUTEROL 2-4 PUFFS INITIALLY, MAY REPEAT AFTER 10-20 MINUTES**
	→	**ADMINISTER OXYGEN**
	→	**ACTIVATE EMS - CALL FOR ASSISTANCE IF PATIENT'S CONDITION DETERIORATES**
	→	**CHECK PATIENT'S RECORD FOR MEDICATIONS, FREQUENCY AND SEVERITY OF ATTACKS**

SIGNS WHEN PATIENT IS RECOVERING

- Patient's breathing returns to normal rate and sound

SIGNS WHEN PATIENT IS DETERIORATING

- Breathing does not improve; cyanosis develops; vital signs are unstable; re-evaluate diagnosis

AIRWAY OBSTRUCTION

Cause: *Foreign body in larynx and pharynx*

SYMPTOMS: Choking, gagging, violent expiratory effort, substernal notch retraction, cyanosis, labored breathing, rapid pulse initially then decreased pulse, respiratory arrest, cardiac arrest

TREATMENT:

PATIENT PLACEMENT   →   **SUPINE IF PATIENT LOSES CONSCIOUSNESS, OTHERWISE UPRIGHT OR AS COMFORTABLE FOR PATIENT**

AIRWAY AND BREATHING   →   **IF PATIENT SHOWS UNIVERSAL SIGNS OF CHOKING (ie, definite airway obstruction), PERFORM HEIMLICH MANEUVER; CONTINUE UNTIL CLEAR OR PATIENT LOSES CONSCIOUSNESS**

  →   **OTHERWISE ATTEMPT TO CLEAR AIRWAY (if problem is associated with aspiration of any item or restoration used in a dental procedure); CLEAR MANUALLY OR SUCTION DEBRIS**

IF NO SUCCESS AT CLEARING AIRWAY, AND IF PATIENT LOSES CONSCIOUSNESS:

  →   **ACTIVATE EMS CALL FOR ASSISTANCE**

  →   **PLACE PATIENT SUPINE**

  →   **TILT HEAD BACKWARD AND CONTINUE TO ATTEMPT TO OPEN AIRWAY**

  →   **CHECK FOR RESPIRATORY SOUNDS; VENTILATE IF POSSIBLE**

  →   **PERFORM ABDOMINAL THRUSTS**

ADVANCED TRAINING ONLY:

  →   **Use laryngoscope; if obstruction is visible, try to dislodge using McGill forcep**

  →   **Perform cricothyrotomy, if unable to clear airway**

SIGNS WHEN PATIENT IS RECOVERING

- Breathing returns to normal; foreign body is removed or swallowed*

SIGNS WHEN PATIENT IS DETERIORATING

- Cyanosis becomes obvious; patient loses consciousness; cardiac or respiratory arrest; re-evaluate diagnosis; maintain basic life support (see pages 13-15); await EMS

*IF THE FOREIGN BODY IS NOT RECOVERED OR PASSES, REFER PATIENT AS SOON AS POSSIBLE FOR RADIOGRAPHIC LOCALIZATION.

CHEST PAIN

MOST COMMON

Angina Pectoris

Acute Myocardial Infarction (AMI) / Heart Attack

**Changes in rhythm, pulse, or blood pressure
may accompany of the cardiovascular states and
should be monitored as part of the
Basic Action Plan for Stabilization
and compared to baseline.**

**Prolonged dysfunction of heart rhythm or blood
pressures mandates immediate emergency
medical transport to a hospital.**

Tachycardia (rapid pulse) — Syncope (fainting), airway obstruction (initially only), epinephrine reactions, adrenal insufficiency, myocardial infarction, thyrotoxicosis, panic attack, hypertension

Decreased blood pressure — Syncope (fainting), postural hypotension, anaphylactic shock, cardiac arrest, allergic drug reactions

Bradycardia — Drug overdose / epinephrine interactions

ANGINA PECTORIS

Cause: Insufficient blood supply to cardiac muscle; may be precipitated by stress and anxiety

SYMPTOMS: Pain in chest, vitals signs satisfactory, patient history of angina (pain persists 3-5 minutes). **Refer to the following page for additional information**

TREATMENT:

PATIENT PLACEMENT	→	UPRIGHT / SEMI-RECLINING
AIRWAY AND BREATHING	→	ADMINISTER OXYGEN
CIRCULATION	→	MONITOR PULSE
	→	PROCEED WITH CPR IF NECESSARY
ADDITIONAL MANAGEMENT	→	IF UNSURE, CONSIDER ACTIVATING EMS IMMEDIATELY
	→	CHECK PATIENT'S RECORD FOR HISTORY AND MEDICATIONS
	→	IF NO HISTORY OF ANGINA OR IF PATIENT HAS A HISTORY OF ANGINA, BUT THIS EPISODE IS NOT TYPICAL OR IF PAIN DOES NOT SUBSIDE WITH NITROGLYCERIN, TREAT AS MYOCARDIAL INFARCTION AND ACTIVATE EMS IMMEDIATELY
	→	ADMINISTER NITROGLYCERIN 0.2-0.6 mg SUBLINGUALLY, MAY BE REPEATED IN 5 MINUTES, UP TO 3 TIMES OVER 15 MINUTES PROVIDED SYSTOLIC BLOOD PRESSURE REMAINS >100
	→	MONITOR VITAL SIGNS
	→	REASSURE PATIENT; REFER FOR EMERGENT MEDICAL RE-EVALUATION IF ANGINA ATTACKS ARE BECOMING MORE FREQUENT
	→	ACTIVATE EMS CALL FOR ASSISTANCE IF PATIENT'S CONDITION DETERIORATES

SIGNS WHEN PATIENT IS RECOVERING

- Pain subsides; vital signs remain stable

SIGNS WHEN PATIENT IS DETERIORATING

- Pain does not subside; vital signs are unstable; re-evaluate diagnosis as likely AMI

ANGINA PECTORIS — SIGNS AND SYMPTOMS

- Early symptoms are often mistaken for indigestion

- As an attack worsens, pain originates behind sternum and radiates to:
  - either of the upper extremities (usually the left) with pain radiating to the shoulder, arm, and elbow (in some cases the pain may extend down the limb to the little finger)
  - neck, jaws, and teeth
  - upper back
  - superior, medial abdomen

- Pain may not originate under the sternum

- Some patients have pain only in the jaw or the teeth

- Shortness of breath

- Nausea

- Pain lasts throughout attack and is not influenced by movement, breathing, or coughing

- Pain usually lasts 3-5 minutes

- Pain diminishes when physical or emotional stress ends

- Patient usually remains still

EMERGENCY CARE

- Any angina pectoris attack is only stable, and therefore, treatable in the dental office, if the episode is typical for the patient (ie, pain is just like every other episode) and responds similarly to nitroglycerin.

- Provide emotional support

- Supply oxygen at a high flow rate (15 L/minute) through a nonrebreather mask

- Place the patient in a restful, comfortable position

- Assist the patient with medication (nitroglycerin)

WARNING!

If there is any doubt regarding differentiation
of angina pectoris and AMI, activate EMS and treat for AMI!

ACUTE MYOCARDIAL INFARCTION

Cause: Occlusion of coronary vessels

SYMPTOMS: Severe pain in chest which may radiate to neck, shoulder, and jaws (if history of angina, may not respond to nitroglycerin); palpitations, tachycardia; pulse thready; dyspnea; cyanosis; diaphoresis; weakness; feeling of impending doom

**IF AMI APPEARS TO BE THE CONDITION,
ACTIVATE EMERGENCY MEDICAL CALL FOR ASSISTANCE IMMEDIATELY!**

TREATMENT:

PATIENT PLACEMENT	→	**UPRIGHT / SEMI-RECLINING OR AS**
AIRWAY AND BREATHING	→	**ACTIVATE EMS, PROCEED WITH BASIC LIFE SUPPORT, ADMINISTER OXYGEN NASAL CANNULA (4-6 L/minute flow rate) OR WITH FACE MASK (15 L/minute)**
CIRCULATION	→	**MONITOR PULSE**
	→	**PROCEED WITH CPR ONLY IF PATIENT SHOWS SIGNS OF CARDIAC ARREST**
ADDITIONAL MANAGEMENT	→	**MONITOR VITAL SIGNS**
	→	**ADMINISTER NITROGLYCERIN 0.2-0.6 mg SUBLINGUALLY, MAY BE REPEATED IN 5 MINUTES, UP TO 3 TIMES OVER 15 MINUTES PROVIDED SYSTOLIC BLOOD PRESSURE REMAINS >100**
	→	**IF PATIENT IS NOT ALLERGIC TO ASPIRIN, ADMINISTER ASPIRIN 160-325 mg (chewed and absorbed in mouth)**
	→	**REASSURE PATIENT, PROCEED WITH BLS PROCEDURES IF PATIENT LOSES CONSCIOUSNESS**
	→	**IF TRAINED, and if patient does not respond to 3 doses of nitroglycerin, administer morphine sulfate 2-4 mg I.V.**

MANAGEMENT OF SPECIAL COMPLICATIONS

- **Arrhythmias: Do not administer drugs unless EKG is on site**
- Sudden death: Administer BLS (see pages 13-15)
- Transfer to hospital; accompany patient in ambulance if possible

SIGNS WHEN PATIENT IS RECOVERING

- Patient appears stable; pain lessens; need for transport to hospital **still necessary**

SIGNS WHEN PATIENT IS DETERIORATING

- Cardiac or respiratory arrest; loss of consciousness; CPR fails

ACUTE MYOCARDIAL INFARCTION (AMI) - SIGNS AND SYMPTOMS

Respiratory
Dyspnea, shallow or deep respirations
Cough that produces frothy, pink sputum

Circulatory
Increased or decreased pulse rate, sometimes irregular
Elevator or reduced blood pressure

Behavioral
Anxiety, irritability, inability to concentrate
Depression
Feeling of impending doom
Mild delirium, personality changes
Fainting
Occasional thrashing about and chest-pounding

Pain
Marked discomfort, continues when at rest
Compressing, constricting, or aching pain rather than a sharp or throbbing pain; may also be described as indigestion
Usually not alleviated by nitroglycerin
May last several minutes
Originates under sternum and may radiate to arms, neck, or jaw

EMERGENCY CARE

Unconscious Patient
Establish and maintain an airway and activate EMS
Provide pulmonary resuscitation or CPR
Administer high concentration of oxygen
Transport immediately
If patient develops respirator or cardiac arrest, deliver oxygen with a bag-valve mask unit or a demand-valve resuscitator

Conscious Patient
Keep the patient calm and still
Take history and determine vital signs
Help patient with medications
Administer high concentration of oxygen
Conserve patient's body heat
Transport as soon as possible in a semireclining or sitting position
Monitor vital signs during transport

Emergency care may be complicated by many factors. If the patient is conscious, his/her irritability, restlessness, and feeling of impending doom may make him/her uncooperative and unwilling to settle down, even though it is vital that the patient does so. Oxygen can be delivered via nasal cannula or face mask (15 L/minute), but many patients will resist the placement of a face mask for oxygen delivery. If the patient resists after an explanation of the importance of oxygen, use a nasal cannula at 4-6 L/minute. Provide needed oxygen, but do not upset the patient.

DISTINGUISHING BETWEEN ANGINA AND ACUTE MYOCARDIAL INFARCTION (AMI)

ANGINA PECTORIS
- Pain follows exertion or stress
- Pain relieved by rest
- Pain usually relieved by nitroglycerin
- Pain lasts 3-5 minutes
- Not associated with arrhythmias
- Blood pressure usually not affected

AMI
- Pain often related to stress or exertion, but may occur at rest
- Rest usually does not relieve pain
- Nitroglycerin may relieve pain briefly, but pain returns
- Pain lasts 30 minutes to several hours
- Often associated with arrhythmias
- Blood pressure is often reduced, but many patients have "normal" BP

WARNING!

If there is any doubt regarding differentiation of angina pectoris and AMI, activate EMS and treat for AMI!

ALLERGIC DRUG REACTIONS

MOST COMMON ALLERGIC REACTIONS

Urticaria or Pruritus

Anaphylactic Shock

MOST COMMON DRUG REACTIONS

Epinephrine Reaction

Drug Overdoses

URTICARIA OR PRURITUS

Cause: Allergy

SYMPTOMS: Urticaria (red eruption on face, neck, hands, and arms), pruritus (itching of these areas)

TREATMENT:

PATIENT PLACEMENT → **UPRIGHT / SEMI-RECLINING**

AIRWAY AND BREATHING → **ADMINISTER OXYGEN**

CIRCULATION → **MONITOR PULSE**

ADDITIONAL MANAGEMENT → **IF UNSURE, CONSIDER ACTIVATING EMS IMMEDIATELY**

→ **MONITOR VITAL SIGNS**

→ **WITHDRAW DRUG IN QUESTION**

→ **ADMINISTER BENADRYL®** (diphenhydramine hydrochloride) 25-50 mg orally; more severe reaction and if trained: ADMINISTER **BENADRYL®** (diphenhydramine hydrochloride) 25-50 mg I.V. or I.M. initially

→ **EPINEPHRINE IS SELDOM NECESSARY, BUT IF REACTION APPEARS SEVERE, ACTIVATE EMS AND ADMINISTER EPINEPHRINE 0.3-0.5 mL (1:1000 solution) SubQ, or I.M.****

NOTE: I.V. administration is generally not utilized unless cardiac monitoring is available and is used only in severe reactions (true anaphylaxis): 0.1 mg (1:10,000 solution) I.V. over 5 minutes. Severe airway obstruction and persistent hypotension requires I.V. use.

**Injection into the floor of the mouth (sublingual) mucosa has been suggested as an alternative route when significant hypotension and reduced perfusion may delay uptake from the conventional I.M. route and I.V. access is not attainable.

→ **AS FOLLOW-UP, PRESCRIBE ORAL ANTIHISTAMINES**
Diphenhydramine: 25-50 mg every 6-8 hours for 3 days

→ **ACTIVATE EMS – CALL FOR ASSISTANCE IF PATIENT'S CONDITION DETERIORATES**

SIGNS WHEN PATIENT IS RECOVERING

- Symptoms subside

SIGNS WHEN PATIENT IS DETERIORATING

- Eruptions / symptoms worsen; signs similar to anaphylaxis appear with respiratory distress; re-evaluate diagnosis

MEDICATIONS WITH ELEVATED INCIDENCE OF HYPERSENSITIVITY REACTIONS

HYPERSENSITIVITY / ALLERGIC REACTIONS >10%

Ampicillin
Asparaginase
Brimonidine
Melphalan

Neomycin, polymyxin B, and
  hydrocortisone
Paclitaxel
Pegaspargase

Streptokinase
Sulfadoxine and pyrimethamine
Trimethoprim and sulfamethoxazole
Urokinase

HYPERSENSITIVITY / ALLERGIC REACTIONS 1% to 10% (MOST COMMON DRUGS)

Amlexanox
Anistreplase
Bacitracin and polymyxin B
Bacitracin, neomycin, and polymyxin B
Butalbital compound and codeine
Cefotetan
Ceftazidime
Cidofovir
Colchicine and probenecid
Cyclopentolate
Dalteparin
Dorzolamide
Erythromycin
Erythromycin and sulfisoxazole
Estrogens and medroxyprogesterone

Hydroxyprogesterone caproate
Ifosfamide
Insulin preparations
Lamotrigine
Latanoprost
Leflunomide
Measles virus vaccine, live
Medroxyprogesterone acetate
Megestrol acetate
Methotrexate
Methylphenidate
Microfibrillar collagen hemostat
Norethindrone
Norgestrel
Nystatin and triamcinolone

Pegaspargase
Penicillin G benzathine and procaine,
  combined
Penicillin V potassium
Pilocarpine
Pilocarpine and epinephrine
Prednicarbate
Prednisolone and gentamicin
Progesterone
Teniposide
Thrombin, topical
Tobramycin and dexamethasone
Trastuzumab
Trimetrexate glucuronate

RASH / PRURITUS >10%

Abacavir (children 11%)
Adapalene
Aldesleukin
Allopurinol
Alprazolam
Ampicillin
Ampicillin and probenecid
Atovaquone
Budesonide
Calcipotriene
Chlordiazepoxide
Cidofovir (rash)
Cladribine
Clonazepam
Diclofenac
Etodolac
Fenoprofen (skin rash)
Fludarabine
Flunisolide
Flurazepam
Flurbiprofen

Gemcitabine
Griseofulvin
Halazepam
Hydrocodone and ibuprofen
Idarubicin
Indomethacin
Isotretinoin
Ketoprofen
Levorphanol
Maprotiline
Meclofenamate
Mefenamic acid
Methimazole
Miconazole
Midodrine
Mitotane
Nabumetone
Nevirapine
Nicotine (transdermal)
Oprelvekin
Oxaprozin

Oxyphenbutazone
Pentamidine
Pentostatin (rash)
Pimozide
Piroxicam
Prazepam
Propylthiouracil
Rifabutin
Risedronate
Sulfamethoxazole
Sulindac
Tacrolimus
Tamoxifen
Thalidomide (rash)
Tolmetin
Trastuzumab
Tretinoin, oral
Trimethoprim
Trimethoprim and sulfamethoxazole

For the sake of brevity, the listing of drugs having an elevated incidence of causing urticaria or pruritus has been limited to medications with an incidence of >10%. Many other medications cite such reactions as 1% to 10% incidence; refer to individual drug monographs in Lexi-Comp's Drug Information Handbook for Dentistry for additional information.

ANAPHYLACTIC SHOCK

Cause: Severe allergic reaction (immediate hypersensitivity)

SYMPTOMS: Progressive respiratory and circulatory failure; itching of nose and hands; flushed face; feeling of substernal depression; labored breathing, stridor; coughing; sudden hypotension; cyanosis; loss of consciousness; incontinence. Sometimes local reactions, such as angioneurotic edema, involve swelling of the tongue and oropharynx, and therefore, progress to respiratory distress. For this reason, its treatment should be as though anaphylaxis is occurring.

**IF SUSPICIOUS OF ANAPHYLAXIS, ACTIVATE EMERGENCY MEDICAL
CALL FOR ASSISTANCE IMMEDIATELY!**

TREATMENT:

PATIENT PLACEMENT	→	**SUPINE**
AIRWAY AND BREATHING	→	**ADMINISTER OXYGEN AND VENTILATE MANUALLY IF NECESSARY**
CIRCULATION	→	**MONITOR PULSE AND VITAL SIGNS**
ADDITIONAL MANAGEMENT	→	**CHECK PATIENT'S RECORD FOR HISTORY AND MEDICATIONS TO ADVISE EMT**

→ **ADMINISTER EPINEPHRINE 0.3-0.5 mL** (1:1000 solution) SubQ, I.M.**; monitor vital signs and communicate with the EMT *en route* as to the advisability of additional injection should the patient not respond.

**Injection into the floor of the mouth (sublingual) mucosa has been suggested as an alternative route when significant hypotension and reduced perfusion may delay uptake from the conventional I.M. route and I.V. access is not attainable.

If trained in advanced life support, while awaiting arrival of EMT, consider: I.V. administration is generally not utilized unless cardiac monitoring is available and is used only in severe reactions (true anaphylaxis): 0.1 mg (1:10,000 solution) I.V. over 5 minutes. Severe airway obstruction and persistent hypotension requires I.V. use.

→ **Bronchospasm/laryngospasm:** Administer bronchodilator-mistometer (albuterol 2-4 puffs initially / may repeat after 10-20 minutes)

→ **Moderate to severe anaphylaxis (to prevent late-phase recurrence of symptoms):** Administer Decadron® (dexa-methasone) 4 mg I.V. or hydrocortisone 100 mg I.V. push

→ **Pruritus and/or urticaria:** Administer Benadryl® (diphenhydramine hydrochloride) 25-50 mg I.M. or I.V. (oral route may be used in less severe conditions, but response may be delayed)

→ **START I.V. FLUIDS** (1000 mL of normal saline)

→ **TRANSFER PATIENT TO HOSPITAL VIA EMS**

SIGNS WHEN PATIENT IS DETERIORATING

- Loss of consciousness, breathing unstable

EPINEPHRINE REACTION

SYMPTOMS: Rapid elevation in blood pressure; epinephrine interactions with several drug groups (tricyclic antidepressants and nonselective beta-adrenergic receptor blockers) have been associated with hypertensive episodes.

PATIENT PLACEMENT   ⟶   **POSITION FOR PATIENT COMFORT**

AIRWAY AND BREATHING   ⟶   **ADMINISTER OXYGEN**

ADDITIONAL MANAGEMENT   ⟶   **REASSURE PATIENT**

⟶ **MONITOR VITAL SIGNS; MAY TAKE UP TO 20 MINUTES FOR BLOOD PRESSURE TO RETURN TO NORMAL RANGE**

⟶ **ACTIVATE EMS IF ANY OTHER SIGNS OR SYMPTOMS (eg, arrhythmias) OR IF BLOOD PRESSURE DOES NOT SOON RETURN TO NORMAL**

SEE REVERSE OF THIS PAGE FOR MANAGEMENT OF DRUG OVERDOSES

LOCAL ANESTHETICS

SYMPTOMS: *Excitement of central nervous system followed by depression (rare except in children and small adults); apprehension, restlessness, tremors, rapid pulse, anxiety, confusion, rapid breathing; may lead to seizures*

MANAGEMENT:

<u>Mild Reaction</u>

- Administer oxygen
- Monitor vital signs

<u>Severe Reaction</u>

- Activate emergency medical call for assistance
- Place patient in supine position
- Maintain open airway
- Monitor vital signs
- Manage seizures
- Provide basic life support
- **IF TRAINED, AND IF PATIENT IS IN SEIZURE**, administer anticonvulsant drug, ie, Valium® (diazepam) 5-10 mg I.V. push, not to exceed 5 mg/minute
- Manage postictal state (lethargy following seizure)

SEDATIVE / HYPNOTIC OVERDOSE

SYMPTOMS: *Decreased respiratory rate, cyanosis*

MANAGEMENT:

- Activate emergency medical call for assistance
- Place patient in supine position
- Maintain open airway; administer oxygen and artificially ventilate if no spontaneous respirations
- Monitor vital signs
- If sedation using a benzodiazepine-derived drug results in symptoms of an overdose, flumazenil (Romazicon®) can be given: 0.2 mg I.V. initially, followed by 0.1 mg/minute, up to a total of 1 mg. Otherwise supportive care as outlined above is appropriate until EMT arrives.

Note: Avoid use in patients receiving benzodiazepines on a chronic basis or those with a history of seizures; duration of flumazenil effect [-1 hour] is often shorter than that of most benzodiazepines and patient should be monitored for resedation; it should be also noted that respiratory depression may not be improved, but mental status should improve.

NARCOTIC-ANALGESIC OVERDOSE

SYMPTOMS: *Decreased respiratory rate, cyanosis*

MANAGEMENT:

- Activate emergency medical call for assistance
- Place patient in supine position
- Maintain open airway; administer oxygen and artificially ventilate if patient shows signs of respiratory arrest
- **IF TRAINED,** administer Narcan® (naloxone) 0.4-2 mg I.V.; may be repeated at 2- to 3-minute intervals, not to exceed 10 mg. I.M. or SubQ may be used if I.V. administration is not possible, but response may be delayed.

STROKE / CEREBROVASCULAR ACCIDENT (CVA)

Cause: *Obstruction or hemorrhage of blood vessel of brain*

SYMPTOMS: Sudden onset of numbness or weakness in the face, arm, or leg, especially on one side of the body; confusion or difficulty in talking or understanding speech, trouble seeing in one or both eyes, difficulty with walking, dizziness, or loss of balance and coordination; severe, sudden onset of headache

TRANSPORT PATIENT IMMEDIATELY BY EMS IF AT ALL SUSPICIOUS OF CVA

TREATMENT:

PATIENT PLACEMENT	→	**REFER TO SPECIFIC CONDITION BELOW**
AIRWAY AND BREATHING	→	**ADMINISTER OXYGEN**
CIRCULATION	→	**MONITOR PULSE**
ADDITIONAL MANAGEMENT	→	**CHECK PATIENT'S RECORD FOR HISTORY AND MEDICATIONS**
	→	**MONITOR VITAL SIGNS; AWAIT EMT**

Transient Ischemic Attack (TIA)
(Stroke-like symptoms usually lasting only minutes to an hour but absolutely resolving completely by 24 hours)

- Place patient in upright or semi-reclining position (comfortable for patient)
- Monitor vital signs, administer oxygen
- Refer the patient immediately for medical evaluation and likely admission. Although the symptoms might completely resolve before the patient arrives to the emergency department, they must be strongly encouraged to seek care as TIAs are often warning signs that a person is at increased risk for a more serious and debilitating stroke.

CVA (Conscious Patient)
- Place patient in semi-reclining position
- Monitor vital signs
- Seek medical assistance
- Provide oxygen

CVA (Unconscious Patient)
- Place patient in supine position
- Record vital signs
- Provide basic life support
- Provide oxygen
- Transfer to hospital via EMS

- **Cerebral thrombosis** — Blockage in arteries supplying oxygenated blood will result in damage to affected parts of the brain

- **Cerebral hemorrhage** — Aneurysm or other weakened area of an artery bursts
  Cerebral hemorrhage is often associated with arteriosclerosis and hypertension

  This has two effects:
  - An area of the brain is deprived of oxygenated blood
  - Pooling blood puts increased pressure on the brain, displacing tissue and interfering with function

STROKE / CEREBROVASCULAR ACCIDENT — SIGNS AND SYMPTOMS

- Headache
- Confusion and/or dizziness
- Loss of function of extremities (usually on one side of the body)
- Collapse
- Facial flaccidity and loss of expression
- Impaired speech
- Unequal pupil size
- Rapid, full pulse
- Difficult respiration
- Nausea
- Convulsion
- Coma

EMERGENCY CARE

Unconscious Patient

- Maintain open airway
- Administer oxygen
- Monitor vital signs
- Transport in lateral recumbent position on paralyzed or affected side
- Keep affected limbs underneath patient

Conscious Patient

- Maintain open airway
- Keep patient calm
- Administer oxygen
- Monitor vital signs
- Transport patient in semi-reclining position
- Give nothing by mouth

SEIZURE DISORDERS

Cause: Intermittent disorder of nervous system ,sometimes caused by sudden discharge of cerebral neurons; idiosyncratic reaction to drug

SYMPTOMS: Excitement, tremor, followed by clonic-tonic convulsions; trance-like state

TREATMENT:

PATIENT PLACEMENT	→	**LEAVE PATIENT IN DENTAL CHAIR (SUPINE IS IDEAL)**
AIRWAY AND BREATHING	→	**MAINTAIN OPEN AIRWAY; ADMINISTER OXYGEN BY MASK**
	→	**SUCTION TO HELP KEEP AIRWAY PATENT**
CIRCULATION	→	**MONITOR PULSE**
ADDITIONAL MANAGEMENT	→	**IF UNSURE, CONSIDER ACTIVATING EMS IMMEDIATELY**
	→	**MONITOR VITAL SIGNS**
	→	**LOOSEN CLOTHING, RELOCATE ALL DENTAL INSTRUMENTS AND SUPPLIES, ENSURE SAFETY OF PATIENT**
	→	**BE PREPARED FOR POSTICTAL STATE (LETHARGY FOLLOWING SEIZURE), SUPPORT RESPIRATION**
	→	**ACTIVATE EMS CALL FOR ASSISTANCE IF PATIENT'S CONDITION DETERIORATES**

SIGNS WHEN PATIENT IS RECOVERING

- Patient awakens uninjured

SIGNS WHEN PATIENT IS DETERIORATING

- Injury during convulsive state; loss of consciousness persists; re-evaluate diagnosis

PANIC ATTACK

Cause: Acute anxiety

SYMPTOMS: Chest pain, hyperventilation, anxiety, nausea, vertigo (dizziness), paresthesia (numbness or tingling in extremities), restlessness, trance-like state

TREATMENT:

PATIENT PLACEMENT	→	**POSITION FOR PATIENT COMFORT**
AIRWAY AND BREATHING	→	**DO NOT ADMINISTER OXYGEN IF HYPERVENTILATION IS PART OF THE ATTACK**
CIRCULATION	→	**MONITOR PULSE AND BLOOD PRESSURE**
ADDITIONAL MANAGEMENT	→	**IF UNSURE, CONSIDER ACTIVATING EMS IMMEDIATELY**
	→	**MONITOR VITAL SIGNS**
	→	**ACTIVATE BLS – CALL FOR ASSISTANCE IF PATIENT'S CONDITION DETERIORATES**
	→	**PROCEED WITH CPR ONLY IF NECESSARY**

SIGNS WHEN PATIENT IS RECOVERING

- Patient regains composure

SIGNS WHEN PATIENT IS DETERIORATING

- Patient develops tachycardia; other vital signs appear unstable; re-evaluate diagnosis; cardiac dysfunction must be ruled out; activate EMS if diagnosis is uncertain

SECTION THREE: PROCEDURES AND PROTOCOLS

ANTIBIOTIC PROPHYLAXIS
PREPROCEDURAL GUIDELINES FOR DENTAL PATIENTS

INTRODUCTION

In dental practice, the clinician is often confronted with a decision to prescribe antibiotics. The focus of this section is on the use of antibiotics as a preprocedural treatment in the prevention of adverse infectious sequelae in two commonly encountered situations: Prevention of infective endocarditis and prevention of late infections of prosthetic implants.

The criteria for preprocedural decisions begins with patient evaluation. An accurate and complete medical history is always the initial basis for any prescriptive treatments on the part of the dentist. These prescriptive treatments can include ordering appropriate laboratory tests, referral to the patient's physician for consultation, or an immediate decision to prescribe preprocedural antibiotics. The dentist should also be aware that antibiotic coverage of the patient might be appropriate due to diseases covered elsewhere in this text, such as human immunodeficiency virus, cavernous thrombosis, undiagnosed or uncontrolled diabetes, lupus, renal failure, and periods of neutropenia as are often associated with cancer chemotherapy. In these instances, medical consultation is almost always necessary in making antibiotic decisions in order to tailor the treatment and dosing to the individual patient's needs. When in doubt regarding a patient's medical status, communicating with the physician is always an appropriate and prudent step.

Note: The ADA Council on Scientific Affairs recently restated the dentist's responsibility when prescribing antibiotics to oral contraceptive users (JADA, 2002, 133:880). It is recommended that dental professionals advise these patients to consult their physician for additional barrier contraception due to potential reduction in the efficacy of oral contraceptives from antibiotic interaction.

PREVENTION OF INFECTIVE ENDOCARDITIS

In one of the most significant examples of Evidence Based Science, the American Heart Association (AHA), in conjunction with the American Dental Association (ADA) and other experts in both medicine and dentistry, reviewed the evidence regarding the use of antibiotic prophylaxis to prevent infective endocarditis (IE) prior to dental appointments. The reviewers concluded that IE is more frequently caused by a patient's susceptibility to bacteremias associated with normal activities rather than bacteremia caused by dental procedures. Therefore, maintaining oral health to reduce bacteremia is more effective in reducing the risk of IE than the use of prophylactic antibiotics before dental procedures. Since the mid-1950s, patients at risk for IE from a variety of conditions have been routinely premedicated with antibiotics prior to dental and other procedures. After a review of the evidence, it has been concluded that the majority of patients did not benefit from this prophylaxis. The incidence of IE was not changed when compared to patients who received IE prophylaxis and those who did not and the risk for adverse effects from antibiotic use exceeded the benefit of therapy. Therefore, based on the evidence, a change in the Guidelines has been recommended by AHA, the ADA, as well as the Infectious Disease Society. The AHA/ADA recommends that most patients no longer need short-term antibiotics as a preventive measure before their dental treatment. Only those patients with the highest risk should receive prophylaxis.

Antibiotic prophylaxis with dental procedures is recommended for patients at high risk of IE due to specific cardiac conditions:

- prosthetic cardiac valve

- a prior incidence of IE

- prophylaxis is also required for heart transplant patients who develop cardiac valvulopathy

- patients with congenital heart disease (CHD) are only required prophylaxis with the following conditions:

  - unrepaired cyanotic CHD, including palliative shunts and conduits

  - CHD repaired by prosthetic material or device (for first 6 months after procedure)

  - **or** if there are residual defects after repair (inhibiting endothelialization)

These patients with high-risk cardiac conditions are recommended for prophylaxis for all dental procedures involving manipulation of gingival tissue or the periapical region of teeth or perforation of the oral mucosa.

Dental procedures that do not require prophylaxis include:

- routine anesthetic injection into noninfected tissue
- taking dental radiographs
- placement of removable prosthodontic or orthodontic appliances
- adjustment of orthodontic appliances, placement of orthodontic brackets
- shedding of deciduous teeth
- bleeding from trauma to the lips or oral mucosa

ANTIBIOTIC SELECTION

For examples of sample prescriptions, see Infective Endocarditis (Prevention). The dentist should be vigilant in reviewing literature for updates.

Amoxicillin is an amino-type penicillin with an extended spectrum of antibacterial action compared to penicillin VK. The pharmacology of amoxicillin as a dental antibiotic has been reviewed previously in *General Dentistry*. The suggested regimen for standard general prophylaxis is a dose of 2 g 30-60 minutes before the procedure. A follow-up dose is no longer necessary. The pediatric dose is 50 mg/kg orally 30-60 minutes before the procedure and not to exceed the adult dose. Amoxicillin is available in capsules (250 mg and 500 mg), chewable tablets (125 mg, 200 mg, 250 mg, 400 mg), tablets (500 mg, 875 mg), and liquid suspension (125 mg/5 mL, 200 mg/5 mL, 250 mg/5 mL, 400 mg/5 mL).

For individuals unable to take oral medications, intramuscular or intravenous ampicillin is recommended for both adults and children. It is to be given at the same doses used for the oral amoxicillin medication. Ampicillin is also an amino-type penicillin having an antibacterial spectrum similar to amoxicillin. Ampicillin is not absorbed from the GI tract as effectively as amoxicillin and, therefore, is not recommended for oral use. Cefazolin or ceftriaxone are alternatives.

Table 1.
PROPHYLACTIC REGIMENS FOR INFECTIVE ENDOCARDITIS FOR DENTAL PROCEDURES

Situation	Drug	Single Dosage 30-60 minutes prior to procedure
Oral	Amoxicillin	Children: 50 mg/kg Adults: 2 g
Unable to take oral medications	Ampicillin or	Children: 50 mg/kg I.M. or I.V. Adults: 2 g I.M. or I.V.
	Cefazolin or Ceftriaxone	Children: 50 mg/kg I.M. or I.V. Adults: 1 g I.M. or I.V.
Allergic to penicillins or ampicillin (oral)	Cephalexin[1,2] or	Children: 50 mg/kg Adults: 2 g
	Clindamycin (systemic) or	Children: 20 mg/kg Adults: 600 mg
	Azithromycin (systemic) or Clarithromycin	Children: 15 mg/kg Adults: 500 mg
Allergic to penicillins or ampicillin and unable to take oral medications	Cefazolin or Ceftriaxone[2]	Children: 50 mg/kg I.M. or I.V. Adults: 1 g I.M. or I.V
	Clindamycin (systemic)	Children: 20 mg/kg I.M. or I.V. Adults: 600 mg I.M. or I.V.

Note: Intramuscular injections should be avoided in patients receiving anticoagulant therapy.
[1] Can use first- or second-generation oral cephalosporins in equivalent doses.
[2] Cephalosporins should not be used in individuals with immediate-type hypersensitivity reaction (urticaria, angioedema, or anaphylaxis) to penicillins.

Individuals who are allergic to the penicillins, such as amoxicillin or ampicillin, should be treated with an alternate antibiotic. The new guidelines have suggested a number of alternate agents including clindamycin, cephalosporins, azithromycin, and clarithromycin. Clindamycin (Cleocin®) occupies an important niche in dentistry as a useful and effective antibiotic and it was a recommended alternative agent for the prevention of bacterial endocarditis in the previous guidelines. In the new guidelines, the oral adult dose is 600 mg 30-60 minutes before the procedure. A follow-up dose is not necessary. Clindamycin is available as 300 mg capsules; thus two capsules will provide the recommended dose. The children's oral dose for clindamycin is 20 mg/kg 30-60 minutes before the procedure. Clindamycin is also available as flavored granules for oral solution. When reconstituted with water, each bottle yields a solution containing 75 mg/5 mL. Intravenous clindamycin is recommended in adults and children who are allergic to penicillin and unable to take oral medications.

Clindamycin was developed in the 1960s as a semisynthetic derivative of lincomycin which was found in the soil organism, Streptomyces lincolnensis, near Lincoln, Nebraska. It is commercially available as the hydrochloride salt to improve solubility in the GI tract. Clindamycin is antibacterial against most aerobic gram-positive cocci, including staphylococci and streptococci, and against many types of anaerobic gram-negative and gram-positive organisms. It has been used over the years in dentistry as an alternative to penicillin and erythromycins for the treatment of oral-facial infections.

The mechanism of antibacterial action of clindamycin is the same as erythromycin. It inhibits protein synthesis in susceptible bacteria resulting in the inhibition of bacterial growth and replication. Following oral administration of a single dose of clindamycin (150 mg, 300 mg, or 600 mg) on an empty stomach, 90% of the dose is rapidly absorbed into the bloodstream and peak serum concentrations are attained within 45-80 minutes. Administration with food does not markedly impair absorption into the bloodstream. Clindamycin serum levels exceed the minimum inhibitory concentration (MIC) for bacterial growth for at least 6 hours after the recommended dose of 600 mg. The serum half-life is 2-3 hours.

Adverse effects of clindamycin after a single dose are virtually nonexistent. Although it is estimated that 1% of patients taking clindamycin will develop symptoms of pseudomembranous colitis, these symptoms usually develop after 9-14 days of clindamycin therapy. These symptoms are rare and only one case has been reported in a patient taking an acute dose for the prevention of endocarditis.

In lieu of clindamycin, penicillin-allergic individuals may receive cephalexin (Keflex®) provided that they have not had an immediate-type sensitivity reaction such as anaphylaxis, urticaria, or angioedema to penicillins. These antibiotics are first-generation cephalosporins having an antibacterial spectrum of action similar to amoxicillin and ampicillin. They elicit a bactericidal action by inhibiting cell wall synthesis in susceptible bacteria. The recommended adult prophylaxis dose for either of these drugs is 2 g 30-60 minutes before the procedure. Again, no follow-up dose is needed. The children's oral dose for cephalexin is 50 mg/kg 30-60 minutes before the procedure. Cephalexin is supplied as capsules (250 mg, 500 mg, 750 mg) and is available in the form of powder for oral suspension at concentrations of 125 mg/5 mL and 250 mg/5 mL.

For those individuals (adults and children) allergic to penicillin and unable to take oral medicines, parenteral cefazolin (Ancef®) may be used, provided they do not have the sensitivities described previously. Cefazolin is also a first-generation cephalosporin. Please note that parenteral cefazolin can be given I.M. or I.V. (refer to Table 1, for the adult and children's doses of parenteral cefazolin).

Azithromycin (Zithromax®) and clarithromycin (Biaxin®) are members of the class of antibiotics known as macrolides. The pharmacology of these drugs has been reviewed previously in General Dentistry. Erythromycins have been available for use in dentistry and medicine since the mid 1950s. Azithromycin and clarithromycin represent the first additions to this class in more than 40 years. The adult prophylactic dose for either drug is 500 mg 30-60 minutes before the procedure with no follow-up dose. The pediatric prophylactic dose of azithromycin and clarithromycin is 15 mg/kg orally 30-60 minutes before the procedure. Although the erythromycin family of drugs is known to inhibit the hepatic metabolism of theophylline and carbamazepine to enhance their effects, azithromycin has not been shown to affect the liver metabolism of these drugs.

Azithromycin is well absorbed from the gastrointestinal tract and is extensively taken up from circulation into tissues with a slow release from those tissues. It reaches peak serum levels in 2-4 hours and serum half-life is 68 hours. Zithromax® is supplied as 250 mg, 500 mg, and 600 mg tablets. It is also available for oral suspension at concentrations of 100 mg/5 mL, 200 mg/5 mL, and single-dose packets containing 1 g.

Clarithromycin (Biaxin®) achieves peak plasma concentrations in 3 hours and maintains effective serum concentrations over a 12-hour period. Reports indicate that it probably interacts with theophylline and carbamazepine by elevating the plasma concentrations of the two drugs. Biaxin® is supplied as 250 mg and 500 mg tablets and 500 mg extended release tablets. It is also available as granules for oral suspension at concentrations of 125 mg/5 mL and 250 mg/5 mL.

Clinical Considerations for Dentistry

Patients with a suspicious history of one of the high-risk cardiac conditions, who are in need of an immediate dental procedure, should be prophylaxed with an appropriate antibiotic prior to the procedure(s) until medical evaluation has been completed and the risk level determined. If unanticipated dental risk develops during a procedure in a cardiac at-risk patient, appropriate antibiotics should be given immediately.

If a series of dental procedures is planned, the clinician must judge whether an interval between procedures, requiring prophylaxis, should be scheduled. The literature supports 9- to 14-day intervals as ideal to minimize the risk of emergence of resistant organisms. Since serum levels of the standard amoxicillin dose may be adequate for 6-14 hours depending on the specific organism challenge, the clinician may have to consider the efficacy of a second dose if multiple procedures are planned over the course of a single day.

PREPROCEDURAL ANTIBIOTICS FOR PROSTHETIC IMPLANTS

A significant number of dental patients have had total joint replacements or other implanted prosthetic devices. Prior to performing dental procedures that might induce bacteremia, the dentist must consider the use of antibiotic prophylaxis in these patients. In February 2009, the American Academy of Orthopedic Surgeons released an updated information statement regarding antibiotic prophylaxis for bacteremia in patients with joint replacements. The guidelines are modestly, but significantly, altered from the guidelines released by the Joint Commission of the Academy of Orthopedic Surgeons and the American Dental Association in 1997 and revised in 2003. The American Dental Association is still considering this new 2009 Information Statement; therefore, the reader is advised to be vigilant for updates.

The most important modification, the 2-year rule for need for prophylaxis, has been eliminated. Prophylaxis is now recommended for all patients with joint prostheses; however, the Academy does go on to describe patients who have the highest risk of joint complications associated with bacteremia (see Table 2). The reader should note that ANTIBIOTIC SELECTION, DOSING, AND REGIMENS HAVE NOT CHANGED. Patients with pins, plates, screws, or other orthopedic hardware that are not within a synovial joint are not at increased risk for hematogenous seeding by microorganisms. Therefore, these patients do not require prophylaxis.

In addition, any clinician, including dentists, planning to carry out a procedure with likely associated bacteremia, is advised to consult with the orthopedist whenever there are questions regarding the potential for complications. This information statement is available at http://www.aaos.org/about/papers/advistmt/1033.asp.

Table 2. PATIENTS WITH THE HIGHEST POTENTIAL RISK OF JOINT INFECTION SUBSEQUENT TO BACTEREMIA

All patients with prosthetic joint replacement

Immunocompromised/immunosuppressed patients

Inflammatory arthropathies (eg, rheumatoid arthritis, systemic lupus erythematosus)

Drug-induced immunosuppression

Radiation-induced immunosuppression

Patients with comorbidity (eg, diabetes, obesity, HIV, and smoking)

Previous prosthetic infections

Malnourishment

Hemophilia

HIV infection

Type 1 diabetes mellitus (insulin dependent, IDDM)

Malignancy

Megaprosthesis

Source: February 2009 AAOS Information Statement. Available at http://www.aaos.org/about/papers/advistmt/1033.asp. Original source: American Dental Association; American Academy of Orthopedic Surgeons, "Antibiotic Prophylaxis for Dental Patients With Total Joint Replacements," *J Am Dent Assoc*, 2003, 134(7):895-9.

The use of antibiotics in patients with prosthetic devices, including total joint replacements, has remained controversial because of several issues. Late infections of implanted prosthetic devices have rarely been associated with microbial organisms of oral origin. Secondly, since late infections in such patients are often not reported, data is lacking to substantiate or refute this potential. There is however, general acceptance that patients with acute infections at distant sites such as the oral cavity may be at greater risk of infection of an implanted prosthetic device.

Periodontal disease has been implicated as a distant site infection. Since antibiotics are associated with allergies and other adverse reactions, and because the frequent use of antibiotics may lead to emergence of resistant organisms, any perceived benefit of antibiotic prophylaxis must always be weighed against known risks of toxicity, allergy, or potential microbial resistance.

ANTIBIOTIC REGIMENS

The antibiotic prophylaxis regimens as suggested by the advisory panel are listed in Table 3. These regimens are not exactly the same as those listed in Table 1 (for prevention of endocarditis) and must be reviewed carefully to avoid confusion. Cephalexin or amoxicillin may be used in patients not allergic to penicillin. The selected antibiotic is given as a single 2 g dose 1 hour before the procedure. A follow-up dose is not recommended. Cephalexin (Keflex®) and amoxicillin were described earlier in this section.

Parenteral cefazolin (Ancef®) or ampicillin is the recommended antibiotic for patients unable to take oral medications (see Table 3 for doses). Cefazolin is a first-generation cephalosporin, effective against anaerobes and aerobic gram-positive bacteria. Ampicillin is an aminopenicillin (described earlier). For patients allergic to penicillin, clindamycin is the recommended antibiotic of choice. Clindamycin is active against aerobic and anaerobic streptococci, most staphylococci, the Bacteroides, and the Actinomyces families of bacteria. The recommended oral and parenteral doses of clindamycin in the joint prosthetic patient are listed in Table 3 below.

Table 3.

ANTIBIOTIC REGIMENS FOR PATIENTS WITH PROSTHETIC IMPLANTS

Patients not allergic to penicillin	Cephalexin or amoxicillin	2 g orally 1 hour prior to the procedure
Patients not allergic to penicillin and unable to take oral medications	Cefazolin **or** Ampicillin	1 g I.M. or I.V. 1 hour prior to the procedure / 2 g I.M. or I.V. 1 hour prior to the procedure
Patients allergic to penicillin	Clindamycin	600 mg orally 1 hour prior to dental procedure
Patients allergic to penicillin and unable to take oral medications	Clindamycin	600 mg I.V. 1 hour prior to dental procedure

Clinical Considerations for Dentistry

The frequency of postinsertion infections in patients who have undergone total joint replacement or prosthetic device placement is variable. The most common cause of infection with all devices is found to be from contamination at the time of surgical insertions. The presence of an acute distant infection at a site other than the joint, however, appears to be a risk factor for late infection of these devices. As more evidence and data are collected, these recommendations may be revised; however, it is thought to be prudent for the dental clinician to fully evaluate all patients with respect to history and/or physical findings prior to determining the risk.

If a dental procedure considered to be low risk for bacteremia is performed in a patient at risk for joint complications, and inadvertent bleeding occurs, then an appropriate antibiotic should be given immediately. Although this is not ideal, animal studies suggest that it may be useful. Likewise, in patients where concern exists over joint complications and a medical consultation cannot be immediately obtained, the patient should be treated as though antibiotic coverage is necessary until such time that an appropriate consultation can be completed. The presence of an acute oral infection, in addition to any pre-existing dental conditions, may increase the risk of late infection at the prosthetic joint. Even though most late joint infections are caused by Staphylococcus sp, the risk of bacteremia involving another organism, predominant in an acute infection, may increase the risk of joint infection.

The dentist may also need to consider the question of multiple procedures over a period of time, rescheduling procedures at intervals of 9-14 days is best. The risk of emergence of resistant organisms in patients receiving multiple short-term doses of antibiotics has been shown to be greater than with those receiving antibiotics over longer intervals of time.

FREQUENTLY ASKED QUESTIONS FOR INFECTIVE ENDOCARDITIS (IE) AND PROSTHETIC IMPLANTS

When should we start following the new prevention of IE guidelines?

Immediately, since the latest guidelines as described herein were released in April, 2007.

What should we do for patients who have been premedicated in the past?

Most patients will no longer require premedication. If the patient does not fall into one of the highest risk groups, premedication should be discontinued. If it cannot be clearly determined if the patient is in the highest risk group, a medical consultation should be sent to determine if prophylaxis should be continued.

Are there different drugs and regimens?

The drugs have undergone minor revisions (see Table 1) and the dosing regimens for all drugs has been changed from 1 hour prior to 30-60 minutes prior to procedure.

Should I just premedicate to be safe?

No, the new guidelines are based on evidence which documents that the risk of adverse side effects from the antibiotics (allergy, GI upset, development of microbial resistance, etc) outweigh the benefits in most patients who previously received SBE/IE prophylaxis. The new Guidelines clearly recommend the use of prophylactic antibiotics only for those with the highest risk.

Has there been any change in the Guidelines for prophylaxis for patients with prosthetic joint replacements?

No, continue to use the published Guidelines.

What if a patient did not meet the new high-risk criteria outlined in the new Guidelines and the patient's physician still recommends IE prophylaxis?

Please contact the physician to see if there are compelling medical reasons for continuing IE prophylaxis.

What if a patient who has received IE prophylaxis in the past for a condition that is now deemed as NOT being high risk for IE prophylaxis still insists on being premedicate?

Recommend that the patient contacts the physician to see if there are compelling medical reasons for continuing IE prophylaxis.

If the patient is presently taking antibiotics for some other ailment, is prophylaxis still necessary?

If a patient is already taking antibiotics for another condition, prophylaxis (when deemed necessary under the new guidelines) should be accomplished with a drug from another class. For example, in the patient who is not allergic to penicillin who is taking a macrolide antibiotic for a medical condition, such as Mycoplasma infection, amoxicillin would be the drug of choice for prophylaxis. Also, in the penicillin-allergic patient taking clindamycin, prophylaxis would best be accomplished with azithromycin or clarithromycin.

Can clindamycin be used safely in patients with gastrointestinal disorders?

If a patient has a history of inflammatory bowel disease and is allergic to penicillin, azithromycin or clarithromycin should be selected over clindamycin. In patients with a negative history of inflammatory bowel disease, clindamycin has not been shown to induce colitis following a single-dose administration.

Why do the suggested drug regimens for patients with joint prostheses resemble so closely the regimens for the prevention of endocarditis?

Bacteremia is the predisposing risk factor for the development of endocarditis in those patients at high risk due to a cardiac condition. Likewise, the potential of bacteremia during dental procedures is considered to be the risk factor in some late-joint prostheses infections, even though this risk is presumed to be much lower.

● *How do we determine those patients who have had joint replacement complications?*

Patients who have had complications during the initial placement of a total joint would be those who had infection following placement, those with recurrent pain, or those who have had previous joint replacement failures. If the patient reports even minor complications, a medical consultation with the orthopedist would be the most appropriate action for the dentist.

Is prophylaxis required in patients with pins, screws, or plates often used in orthopedic repairs?

There is currently no evidence supporting use of antibiotics following the placement of pins, plates, or screws. Breast implants, dental implants, and implanted lenses in the eye following cataract surgery are also all thought to be at minimal risk for infection following dental procedures. Therefore, no antibiotic prophylaxis is recommended in these situations. There is, however, some evidence indicating elevated risk of infection following some types of penile implants and some vascular access devices, used during chemotherapy. It is recommended that the dentist discuss such patients with the physician prior to determining the need for antibiotics.

What should I do if medical consultation results in a recommendation that differs from the published guidelines endorsed by the American Dental Association?

The dentist is ultimately responsible for treatment recommendations. Ideally, by communicating with the physician, a consensus can be achieved that is either in agreement with the guidelines or is based on other established medical reasoning.

What is the best antibiotic modality for treating dental infections?

Penicillin is still the drug of choice for treatment of infections in and around the oral cavity. Phenoxymethyl penicillin (Pen VK®) has long been the most commonly selected antibiotic. In penicillin-allergic individuals, erythromycin may be an appropriate consideration. If another drug is sought, clindamycin prescribed 300 mg as a loading dose followed by 150 mg 4 times/day would be an appropriate regimen for a dental infection. In general, if there is no response to Pen VK®, then Augmentin® may be a good alternative in the nonpenicillin-allergic patient because of its slightly altered spectrum. Recommendations would include that the patient take the drug with food.

Is there cross-allergenicity between the cephalosporins and penicillin?

The incidence of cross-allergenicity is 5% to 8% in the overall population. If a patient has demonstrated a Type I hypersensitivity reaction to penicillin, namely urticaria or anaphylaxis, then this incidence would increase to 20%.

Is there definitely an interaction between contraception agents and antibiotics?

There are well-founded interactions between contraceptives and antibiotics. The best instructions that a patient could be given by his/her dentist are that should an antibiotic be necessary, and the dentist is aware that the patient is on contraceptives, and if the patient is using chemical contraceptives, the patient should seriously consider additional means of contraception during the antibiotic management.

Are antibiotics necessary in diabetic patients?

In the management of diabetes, control of the diabetic status is the key factor relative to all morbidity issues. If a patient is well controlled, then antibiotics will likely not be necessary; however, in patients where the control is questionable or where they have recently been given a different drug regimen for their diabetes or if they are being titrated to an appropriate level of either insulin or oral hypoglycemic agents during these periods of time, the dentist might consider preprocedural antibiotics to be efficacious.

Do nonsteroidal anti-inflammatory drugs (NSAIDs) interfere with blood pressure medication?

At the current time there is no clear evidence that NSAIDs interfere with any of the blood pressure medications that are currently in use.

Some materials in this chapter were adapted from the guidelines of Wilson W, Taubert KA, Gewitz M, et al, "Prevention of Infective Endocarditis: Guidelines From the American Heart Association: A Guideline From the American Heart Association Rheumatic Fever, Endocarditis, and Kawasaki Disease Committee, Council on Cardiovascular Disease in the Young, and the Council on Clinical Cardiology, Council on Cardiovascular Surgery and Anesthesia, and the Quality of Care and Outcomes Research Interdisciplinary Working Group," *Circulation*, 2007, 116(15):1736-54.

PROBIOTICS TO REDUCE GASTRIC SYMPTOMS DURING LONG-TERM ANTIBIOTIC THERAPY

Cultures of direct-fed microorganisms or probiotics are able to multiply in the intestinal tract to create a balance of microflora. Some lactobacillus species used in probiotic applications include *L. acidophilus*, *L. casei*, *L. reuteri*, *L. rhamnosus*, and *Bifidobacterium bifidum*. These and other organisms form a symbiotic or mutual relationship with their host. Each species develops a resistance to the disease-causing potential of such organisms and form mutual beneficial relationships with these organisms. The familiar *L. acidophilus* produces lactic acid, reduces gut pH, and acts as a colonizer. Some forms of antibiotics, such as cephalosporins, clindamycin, or fluoroquinolones, induce colitis, an inflammation of the large intestine, in some individuals. This type of colitis is caused by a toxin produced by the bacteria *Clostridium difficile*, which is resistant to many antibiotics and proliferates in the intestines when other normal bacterial flora in the intestine are altered by the antibiotics.

It is usually recommended to take probiotics at least 3 hours apart from antibiotics. Taking both at the same time defeats the purpose as the friendly bacteria will be totally destroyed by the drug. During antibiotic therapy, a good dose of viable probiotic cells is 6-25 billion colony-forming units per day. Probiotics are also being studied as adjunctive therapy to periodontal treatment and treatment of other bacterial infections.

● OXYGEN DELIVERY

The most frequently used drug in the management of medical emergencies is oxygen. Oxygen in tanks is produced by fractional distillation and stored in the tanks under pressure at 2000 PSI. A flow regulator reduces the PSI to a safe range for delivery to the patients.

SAFETY PRECAUTIONS FOR OXYGEN USE

— Never use combustibles in the presence of oxygen, including petroleum products (Vaseline®).

— Do not store oxygen in temperatures >120°F.

— Never adjust the regulator with body directly over the tank.

— Connect the tubing to the tank and adjust the regulator before placing the delivery system onto the patient's face.

— Do not deliver high concentrations of oxygen to patients with chronic obstructive pulmonary disease (COPD)- it removes their remaining stimulus to breathe, the hypoxic drive.

Oxygen cylinder

Should be a Series E held upright in a portable carriage

— Having oxygen in conjunction with nitrous oxide in each operatory does not prepare one to deliver oxygen to patients in the reception area or elsewhere in the office. Therefore, **portable oxygen tanks are a must!**

— A single tank of oxygen may not last until EMS arrives. Therefore, a **back-up tank of oxygen is a must!**

It is constructed of steel or aluminum and contains compressed oxygen under 2000 PSI pressure.

It is color-coded green to differentiate it from other cylinders of compressed gas.

It has a yoke with a 5 pin index which is a system that also differentiates each tank of compressed gas so that only gas-specific delivery systems can be fitted to each respective tank.

Pressure Regulator (Reducing Valve)

Fits the yoke of the oxygen tank, as it has the compatible pin index.

Reduces the pressure of the oxygen flow from the 2000 PSI to levels of 40-70 PSI for safe delivery in administration of oxygen to patients.

Positive pressure devices (demand valve resuscitators) deliver the oxygen at approximately 60 L/minute in short bursts.

— This is designed for delivering intermittent jets of oxygen to patients who are not spontaneously breathing.

— To deliver oxygen to spontaneously breathing patients, the flow rate should be 4-15 L/minute. This requires a flow regulator.

Combination Pressure Regulator

This is the regulator that should be attached to the portable Series E tank in a dental office as it permits delivery of oxygen at low flow rates for medical emergencies and/or supplemental oxygen for asthmatic patients during dental treatment. Unfortunately, many dental offices do not have oxygen tanks with low flow regulators as they are not familiar with them and the need for low delivery of oxygen in medical emergencies.

Contains one spigot for positive pressure (demand valve) which overrides the low flow regulator and delivers the 60 L/minute bursts of oxygen.

Contains another spigot for low-flow delivery at flow rates of 4-15 L/minute for spontaneously breathing patients.

Contains a flow meter to control the rate of oxygen flow.

Oxygen Delivery Systems

Nasal cannula — delivers low to moderate amounts of oxygen to spontaneously breathing patients

Simple face mask — delivers slightly higher concentrations of oxygen than the nasal cannula, but is not as easily tolerated as the nasal cannula

Nonrebreather mask — has a reservoir bag filled with 100% oxygen. A one-way valve from the mask to the reservoir prevents exhaled air from diluting the oxygen concentration and increases the concentration of oxygen inhaled by the patient. The nonrebreathing mask is the best way to deliver high concentrations of oxygen to spontaneously breathing patients.

Bag-valve mask — is used to ventilate patients in CPR and also to assist ventilations in semi-conscious patients in respiratory depression. The bag-valve-mask may be used in atmospheric air ventilation at 21% oxygen or it may be connected to the oxygen tank to deliver concentrations of oxygen from 40% to 100% depending on the valve system and reservoir bag set-up.

Demand valve — has a push button valve connected to a face mask which has a tubing connecting it to the positive pressure spigot. When the button is pressed, a burst of oxygen is released at a very high flow rate (100-150 L/minute). Then, when the operator releases the button, a present pressure (40-50 mm Hg) is set and the flow ceases. This is a safety precaution to prevent overinflating the lungs. So, as the patient's lungs inflate, the pressure within them increases and the oxygen automatically stops. The patient receives oxygen on demand. The device is used to resuscitate patients who are not breathing and to assist ventilations in patients who are in respiratory distress and barely breathing.

Oxygen Delivery Systems

Device	Indications	Flow Rate	Oxygen Delivery
Cannula	Patient is breathing and needs low levels of oxygen	2-6 L/min	25%-40%
Face Mask	Patient is breathing and needs moderate levels of oxygen: – when cannula is not tolerated – when more oxygen is desired – patient is in shock	8-15 L/min	60%
Nonrebreather Mask	Patient is breathing and needs high level of oxygen: – patient is in shock – when more oxygen is needed	10-15 L/min	60%-90%
Bag-Valve Mask	Patient has stopped breathing; used instead of mouth-to-mouth resuscitation.	10-15 L/min	90%-100%

PHOTOCOPY, LAMINATE, AND AFFIX TO THE OXYGEN TANK

OCCUPATIONAL EXPOSURE TO BLOODBORNE PATHOGENS
(STANDARD / UNIVERSAL PRECAUTIONS)

OVERVIEW AND REGULATORY CONSIDERATIONS

Every healthcare employee, from nurse to housekeeper, has some (albeit small) risk of exposure to HIV and other viral agents such as hepatitis B and Jakob-Creutzfeldt agent. The incidence of HIV-1 transmission associated with a percutaneous exposure to blood from an HIV-1 infected patient is approximately 0.3% per exposure. 1 In 1989, it was estimated that 12,000 United States healthcare workers acquired hepatitis B annually. 2 An understanding of the appropriate procedures, responsibilities, and risks inherent in the collection and handling of patient specimens is necessary for safe practice and is required by Occupational Safety and Health Administration (OSHA) regulations.

The Occupational Safety and Health Administration published its "Final Rule on Occupational Exposure to Bloodborne Pathogens" in the Federal Register on December 6, 1991. OSHA has chosen to follow the Centers for Disease Control (CDC) definition of universal precautions. The Final Rule provides full legal force to universal precautions and requires employers and employees to treat blood and certain body fluids as if they were infectious. The Final Rule mandates that healthcare workers must avoid parenteral contact and must avoid splattering blood or other potentially infectious material on their skin, hair, eyes, mouth, mucous membranes, or on their personal clothing. Hazard abatement strategies must be used to protect the workers. Such plans typically include, but are not limited to, the following:

- safe handling of sharp items ("sharps") and disposal of such into puncture-resistant containers

- gloves required for employees handling items soiled with blood or equipment contaminated by blood or other body fluids

- provisions of protective clothing when more extensive contact with blood or body fluids may be anticipated (eg, surgery, autopsy, or deliveries)

- resuscitation equipment to reduce necessity for mouth-to-mouth resuscitation

- restriction of HIV- or hepatitis B-exposed employees to noninvasive procedures

OSHA has specifically defined the following terms: Occupational exposure means reasonably anticipated skin, eye mucous membrane, or parenteral contact with blood or other potentially infectious materials that may result from the performance of an employee's duties. Other potentially infectious materials are human body fluids including semen, vaginal secretions, cerebrospinal fluid, synovial fluid, pleural fluid, pericardial fluid, peritoneal fluid, amniotic fluid, saliva in dental procedures, and body fluids that are visibly contaminated with blood, and all body fluids in situations where it is difficult or impossible to differentiate between body fluids; any unfixed tissue or organ (other than intact skin) from a human (living or dead); and HIV-containing cell or tissue cultures, organ cultures, and HIV- or HBV-containing culture medium or other solutions, and blood, organs, or other tissues from experimental animals infected with HIV or HBV. An exposure incident involves specific eye, mouth, other mucous membrane, nonintact skin, or parenteral contact with blood or other potentially infectious materials that results from the performance of an employee's duties. 3 It is important to understand that some exposures may go unrecognized despite the strictest precautions.

A written Exposure Control Plan is required. Employers must provide copies of the plan to employees and to OSHA upon request. Compliance with OSHA rules may be accomplished by the following methods.

- **Universal precautions (UPs)** means that all human blood and certain body fluids are treated as if known to be infectious for HIV, HBV, and other bloodborne pathogens. UPs do not apply to feces, nasal secretions, saliva, sputum, sweat, tears, urine, or vomitus unless they contain visible blood.

- **Engineering controls (ECs)** are physical devices which reduce or remove hazards from the workplace by eliminating or minimizing hazards or by isolating the worker from exposure. Engineering control devices include sharps disposal containers, self-resheathing syringes, etc.

- **Work practice controls (WPCs)** are practices and procedures that reduce the likelihood of exposure to hazards by altering the way in which a task is performed. Specific examples are the prohibition of two-handed recapping of needles, prohibition of storing food alongside potentially contaminated material, discouragement of pipetting fluids by mouth, encouraging handwashing after removal of gloves, safe handling of contaminated sharps, and appropriate use of sharps containers.

- **Personal protective equipment (PPE)** is specialized clothing or equipment worn to provide protection from occupational exposure. PPE includes gloves, gowns, laboratory coats (the type and characteristics will depend upon the task and degree of exposure anticipated), face shields or masks, and eye protection. Surgical caps or hoods and/or shoe covers or boots are required in instances in which gross contamination can reasonably be anticipated (eg, autopsies, orthopedic surgery). If PPE is penetrated by blood or any contaminated material, the item must be removed immediately or as soon as feasible. **The employer must provide and launder or dispose of all PPE at no cost to the employee.** Gloves must be worn when there is a reasonable anticipation of hand contact with potentially infectious material, including a patient's mucous membranes or nonintact skin. Disposable gloves must be changed as soon as possible after they become torn or punctured. Hands must be washed after gloves are removed. OSHA has revised the PPE standards, effective July 5, 1994, to include the requirement that the employer certify in writing that it has conducted a hazard assessment of the workplace to determine whether hazards are present that will necessitate the use of PPE. Also, verification that the employee has received and understood the PPE training is required. 4

Housekeeping protocols: OSHA requires that all bins, cans, and similar receptacles, intended for reuse which have a reasonable likelihood for becoming contaminated, be inspected and decontaminated immediately or as soon as feasible upon visible contamination and on a regularly scheduled basis. Broken glass that may be contaminated must not be picked up directly with the hands. Mechanical means (eg, brush, dust pan, tongs, or forceps) must be used. Broken glass must be placed in a proper sharps container.

Employers are responsible for teaching appropriate clean-up procedures for the work area and personal protective equipment. A 1:10 dilution of household bleach is a popular and effective disinfectant. It is prudent for employers to maintain signatures or initials of employees who have been properly educated. If one does not have written proof of education of universal precautions teaching, then by OSHA standards, such education never happened.

Pre-exposure and postexposure protocols: OSHA's Final Rule includes the provision that employees, who are exposed to contamination, be offered the hepatitis B vaccine at no cost to the employee. Employees may decline; however, a declination form must be signed. The employee must be offered free vaccine if he/she changes his/her mind. Vaccination to prevent the transmission of hepatitis B in the healthcare setting is widely regarded as sound practice. 5 In the event of exposure, a confidential medical evaluation and follow-up must be offered at no cost to the employee. Follow-up must include collection and testing of blood from the source individual for HBV and HIV if permitted by state law if a blood sample is available. If a postexposure specimen must be specially drawn, the individual's consent is usually required. Some states may not require consent for testing of patient blood after accidental exposure. One must refer to state and/or local guidelines for proper guidance.

The employee follow-up must also include appropriate postexposure prophylaxis, counseling, and evaluation of reported illnesses. The employee has the right to decline baseline blood collection and/or testing. If the employee gives consent for the collection but not the testing, the sample must be preserved for 90 days in the event that the employee changes his/her mind within that time. Confidentiality related to blood testing must be ensured. **The employer does not have the right to know the results** of the testing of either the source individual or the exposed employee.

MANAGEMENT OF HEALTHCARE WORKER EXPOSURES TO HBV, HCV, AND HIV

Adapted from Updated U.S. Public Health Service Guidelines for the Management of Occupational Exposures to HIV and Recommendations for Postexposure Prophylaxis, "Recommended HIV Postexposure Prophylaxis (PEP) for Percutaneous Injuries," *MMWR Recomm Rep*, 2005, 54(RR-9):3-17.

Likelihood of transmission of HIV-1 from occupational exposure is 0.2% per parenteral exposure (eg, needlestick) to blood from HIV-infected patients. Factors that increase risk for occupational transmission include advanced stages of HIV in source patient, hollow bore needle puncture, a poor state of health or inexperience of healthcare worker (HCW). After first aid is initiated, the healthcare worker should report exposure to a supervisor and to the institution's occupational medical service for evaluation. All parenteral exposures should be treated equally until they can be evaluated by the occupational medicine service, who will then determine the actual risk of exposure. Counselling regarding risk of exposure, antiviral prophylaxis, plans for follow up, exposure prevention, sexual activity, and providing emotional support and response to concerns are necessary to support the exposed healthcare worker. Additional information should be provided to healthcare workers who are pregnant or planning to become pregnant.

Immediate actions include aggressive first aid at the puncture site (eg, scrubbing site with povidone-iodine solution or soap and water for 10 minutes) or at mucus membrane site (eg, saline irrigation of eye for 15 minutes), followed by immediate reporting to the hospital's occupational medical service where a thorough investigation should be performed, including identification of the source, type of exposure, volume of inoculum, timing of exposure, extent of injury, appropriateness of first aid, as well as psychological status of the healthcare worker. HIV serologies should be performed on the healthcare worker and HIV risk counselling should begin at this point. Although the data are not clear, antiviral prophylaxis may be offered to healthcare workers who are parenterally or mucous membrane exposed. If used, antiretroviral prophylaxis should be initiated within 1-2 hours after exposure.

Factors to Consider in Assessing the Need for Follow-up of Occupational Exposures

- **Type of Exposure**
  - Percutaneous injury
  - Mucous membrane exposure
  - Nonintact skin exposure
  - Bites resulting in blood exposure to either person involved
- **Type and amount of fluid / tissue**
  - Blood
  - Fluids containing blood
  - Potentially infectious fluid or tissue (semen; vaginal secretions; and cerebrospinal, synovial, pleural, peritoneal, pericardial, and amniotic fluids)
  - Direct contact with concentrated virus
- **Infectious status of source**
  - Presence of HB_sAg
  - Presence of HCV antibody
  - Presence of HIV antibody
- **Susceptibility of exposed person**
  - Hepatitis B vaccine and vaccine response status
  - HBV, HCV, HIV immune status

Evaluation of Occupational Exposure Sources

Known sources

- Test known sources for HBsAg, anti-HCV, and HIV antibody
  - Direct virus assays for routine screening of source patients are not recommended
  - Consider using a rapid HIV-antibody test
  - If the source person is not infected with a blood-borne pathogen, baseline testing or further follow-up of the exposed person is not necessary
- For sources whose infection status remains unknown (eg, the source person refuses testing), consider medical diagnoses, clinical symptoms, and history of risk behaviors
- Do not test discarded needles for blood-borne pathogens

Unknown sources

- For unknown sources, evaluate the likelihood of exposure to a source at high risk for infection
  - Consider the likelihood of blood-borne pathogen infection among patients in the exposure setting

Recommended Postexposure Prophylaxis for Exposure to Hepatitis B Virus

Vaccination and Antibody Response Status of Exposed Workers[1]	Treatment		
	Source HB_sAg[2]-Positive	Source HB_sAg[2]-Negative	Source Unknown or Not Available for Testing
Unvaccinated	HBIG[3] x 1 and initiate HB vaccine series[4]	Initiate HB vaccine series	Initiate HB vaccine series
Previously vaccinated			
Known responder[5]	No treatment	No treatment	No treatment
Known nonresponder[6]	HBIG x 1 and initiate revaccination or HBIG x 2[7]	No treatment	If known high risk source, treat as if source was HBsAg-positive
Antibody response unknown	Test exposed person for anti-HB$_s$[8] 1. If adequate,[5] no treatment is necessary 2. If inadequate,[6] administer HBIG x 1 and vaccine booster	No treatment	Test exposed person for anti-HB$_s$ 1. If adequate,[4] no treatment is necessary 2. If inadequate,[4] administer vaccine booster and recheck titer in 1-2 mos

[1]Persons who have previously been infected with HBV are immune to reinfection and do not require postexposure prophylaxis.
[2]Hepatitis B surface antigen.
[3]Hepatitis B immune globulin; dose is 0.06 mL/kg intramuscularly.
[4]Hepatitis B vaccine.
[5]A responder is a person with adequate levels of serum antibody to HB_sAg (ie, anti-HBs ≥10 mIU/mL).
[6]A nonresponder is a person with inadequate response to vaccination (ie, serum anti-HBs <10 mIU/mL).
[7]The option of giving one dose of HBIG and reinitiating the vaccine series is preferred for nonresponders who have not completed a second 3-dose vaccine series.
For persons who previously completed a second vaccine series but failed to respond, two doses of HBIG are preferred.
[8]Antibody to HB_sAg.

Recommended HIV Postexposure Prophylaxis (PEP) for Percutaneous Injuries

Exposure Type	Infection Status of Source				
	HIV-Positive, Class 1[1]	HIV-Positive, Class 2[1]	Source of Unknown HIV Status[2]	Unknown Source[3]	HIV-Negative
Less severe[4]	Recommend basic 2-drug PEP	Recommend expanded ≥3-drug PEP	Generally, no PEP warranted; however, consider basic 2-drug PEP[5] for source with HIV risk factors[6]	Generally, no PEP warranted; however, consider basic 2-drug PEP[5] in settings in which exposure to HIV-infected persons is likely	No PEP warranted
More severe[7]	Recommend expanded 3-drug PEP	Recommend expanded ≥3-drug PEP	Generally, no PEP warranted; however, consider basic 2-drug PEP[5] for source with HIV risk factors[6]	Generally, no PEP warranted; however, consider basic 2-drug PEP[5] in settings in which exposure to HIV-infected persons is likely	No PEP warranted

[1] HIV-positive, class 1 – asymptomatic HIV infection or known low viral load (eg, <1500 ribonucleic acid copies/mL). HIV-positive, class 2 – symptomatic HIV infection, AIDS, acute seroconversion, or known high viral load. If drug resistance is a concern, obtain expert consultation. Initiation of PEP should not be delayed pending expert consultation, and, because expert consultation alone cannot substitute for face-to-face counseling, resources should be available to provide immediate evaluation and follow-up care for all exposures.
[2] For example, deceased source person with no samples available for HIV testing.
[3] For example, a needle from a sharps disposal container.
[4] For example, solid needle or superficial injury.
[5] The recommendation "consider PEP" indicates that PEP is optional; a decision to initiate PEP should be based on a discussion between the exposed person and the treating clinician regarding the risks versus benefits of PEP.
[6] If PEP is offered and administered and the source is later determined to be HIV-negative, PEP should be discontinued.
[7] For example, large-bore hollow needle, deep puncture, visible blood on device, or needle used in patient's artery or vein.

Recommended HIV Postexposure Prophylaxis (PEP) for Mucous Membrane Exposures and Nonintact Skin[1] Exposures

Exposure Type	Infection Status of Source				
	HIV-Positive, Class 1[2]	HIV-Positive, Class 2[2]	Source of Unknown HIV Status[3]	Unknown Source[4]	HIV-Negative
Small volume[5]	Consider basic 2-drug PEP[6]	Recommend basic 2-drug PEP	Generally, no PEP warranted[7]	Generally, no PEP warranted	No PEP warranted
Large volume[8]	Recommend basic 2-drug PEP	Recommend expanded ≥3-drug PEP	Generally, no PEP warranted; however, consider basic 2-drug PEP[6] for source with HIV risk factors[7]	Generally, no PEP warranted; however, consider basic 2-drug PEP[6] in settings in which exposure to HIV-infected persons is likely	No PEP warranted

[1] For skin exposures, follow-up is indicated only if evidence exists of compromised skin integrity (eg, dermatitis, abrasion, or open wound).
[2] HIV-positive, class 1 – asymptomatic HIV infection or known low viral load (eg, <1500 ribonucleic acid copies/mL). HIV-positive, class 2 – symptomatic HIV infection, AIDS, acute seroconversion, or known high viral load. If drug resistance is a concern, obtain expert consultation. Initiation of PEP should not be delayed pending expert consultation, and, because expert consultation alone cannot substitute for face-to-face counseling, resources should be available to provide immediate evaluation and follow-up care for all exposures.
[3] For example, deceased source person with no samples available for HIV testing.
[4] For example, splash from inappropriately disposed blood.
[5] For example, a few drops.
[6] The recommendation "consider PEP" indicates that PEP is optional; a decision to initiate PEP should be based on a discussion between the exposed person and the treating clinician regarding the risks versus benefits of PEP.
[7] If PEP is offered and administered and the source is later determined to be HIV-negative, PEP should be discontinued.
[8] For example, a major blood splash.

Situations for Which Expert[1] Consultation for HIC Postexposure Prophylaxis Is Advised

- **Delayed (ie, later than 24-36 hours) exposure report**
  - The interval after which there is no benefit from postexposure prophylaxis (PEP) is undefined
- **Unknown source (eg, needle in sharps disposal container or laundry)**
  - Decide use of PEP on a case-by-case basis
  - Consider the severity of the exposure and the epidemiologic likelihood of HIV exposure
  - Do not test needles or sharp instruments for HIV
- **Known or suspected pregnancy in the exposed person**
  - Does not preclude the use of optimal PEP regimens
  - Do not deny PEP solely on the basis of pregnancy
- **Resistance of the source virus to antiretroviral agents**
  - Influence of drug resistance on transmission risk is unknown
  - Selection of drugs to which the source person's virus is unlikely to be resistant is recommended, if the source person's virus is unknown or suspected to be resistant to ≥1 of the drugs considered for the PEP regimen
  - Resistance testing of the source person's virus at the time of the exposure is not recommended

- **Toxicity of the initial PEP regimen**
  - Adverse symptoms, such as nausea and diarrhea, are common with PEP
  - Symptoms can often be managed without changing the PEP regimen by prescribing antimotility and/or antiemetic agents
  - Modification of dose intervals (ie, administering a lower dose of drug more frequently throughout the day, as recommended by the manufacturer), in other situations, might help alleviate symptoms

[1]Local experts and/or the National Clinicians' Postexposure Prophylaxis Hotline (PEPline 1-888-448-4911).

Occupational Exposure Management Resources

National Clinicians' Postexposure Prophylaxis Hotline (PEPline)
Run by University of California-San Francisco/San Francisco General Hospital staff; supported by the Health Resources and Services Administration Ryan White CARE Act, HIV/AIDS Bureau, AIDS Education and Training Centers, and CDC

Phone: (888) 448-4911
Internet: http://www.ucsf.edu/hivcntr

Needlestick!
A website to help clinicians manage and document occupational blood and body fluid exposures. Developed and maintained by the University of California, Los Angeles (UCLA), Emergency Medicine Center, UCLA School of Medicine, and funded in part by CDC and the Agency for Healthcare Research and Quality.

Internet: http://www.needlestick.mednet.ucla.edu

Hepatitis Hotline

hepatitis

Phone: (888) 443-7232
Internet: http://www.cdc.gov/

Reporting to CDC
Occupationally acquired HIV infections and failures of PEP

Phone: (800) 893-0485

HIV Antiretroviral Pregnancy Registry

antiretroviral

Phone: (800) 258-4263
Fax: (800) 800-1052
Address: 1410 Commonwealth Drive, Suite 215
Wilmington, NC 28405
Internet: http://www.glaxowellcome.com/preg_reg/

Food and Drug Administration
Report unusual or severe toxicity to antiretroviral agents

Phone: (800) 332-1088
Address: MedWatch
HF-2, FDA
5600 Fishers Lane
Rockville, MD 20857
Internet: http://www.fda.gov/medwatch

HIV / AIDS Treatment Information Service

Internet: http://www.aidsinfo.nih.gov

Management of Occupational Blood Exposures

Provide immediate care to the exposure site
- Wash wounds and skin with soap and water
- Flush mucous membranes with water

Determine risk associated with exposure by:
- Type of fluid (eg, blood, visibly bloody fluid, other potentially infectious fluid or tissue, and concentrated virus)
- Type of exposure (ie, percutaneous injury, mucous membrane or nonintact skin exposure, and bites resulting in **blood exposure)**

Evaluate exposure source
- Assess the risk of infection using available information
- Test known sources for HB$_s$Ag, anti-HCV, and HIV antibody (consider using rapid testing)
- For unknown sources, assess risk of exposure to HBV, HCV, or HIV infection
- Do not test discarded needle or syringes for virus contamination

Evaluate the exposed person
- Assess immune status for HBV infection (ie, by history of hepatitis B vaccination and vaccine response)

Give PEP for exposures posing risk of infection transmission
- HBV: See Recommended Postexposure Prophylaxis for Exposure to Hepatitis B Virus Table
- HCV: PEP not recommended
- HIV: See Recommended HIV Postexposure Prophylaxis for Percutaneous Injuries Table and Recommended HIV Postexposure Prophylaxis for Mucous Membrane Exposures and Nonintact Skin Exposures Table
  - Initiate PEP as soon as possible, preferably within hours of exposure
  - Offer pregnancy testing to all women of childbearing age not known to be pregnant
  - Seek expert consultation if viral resistance is suspected
  - Administer PEP for 4 weeks if tolerated

Perform follow-up testing and provide counseling
- Advise exposed persons to seek medical evaluation for any acute illness occurring during follow-up

HBV exposures
- Perform follow-up anti-HB$_s$ testing in persons who receive hepatitis B vaccine
  - Test for anti-HBs 1-2 months after last dose of vaccine
  - Anti-HB$_s$ response to vaccine cannot be ascertained if HBIG was received in the previous 3-4 months

HCV exposures
- Perform baseline and follow-up testing for anti-HCV and alanine aminotransferase (ALT) 4-6 months after exposures
- Perform HCV RNA at 4-6 months if earlier diagnosis of HCV infection is desired
- Confirm repeatedly reactive anti-HCV enzyme immunoassays (EIAs) with supplemental tests

HIV exposures
- Perform HIV antibody testing for at least 6 months postexposure (eg, at baseline, 6 weeks, 3 months, and 6 months)
- Perform HIV antibody testing if illness compatible with an acute retroviral syndrome occurs
- Advise exposed persons to use precautions to prevent secondary transmission during the follow-up period
- Evaluate exposed persons taking PEP within 72 hours after exposure and monitor for drug toxicity for at least 2 weeks

Basic and Expanded HIV Postexposure Prophylaxis Regimens

BASIC REGIMENS

Zidovudine (Retrovir®; ZDV; AZT) + lamivudine (Epivir®; 3TC); available as Combivir®

Preferred dosing
- ZDV: 300 mg twice daily or 200 mg three times daily, with food; total: 600 mg daily
- 3TC: 300 mg once daily or 150 mg twice daily
- Combivir®: One tablet twice daily

Dosage forms
- ZDV: 100 mg capsule, 300 mg tablet
- 3TC: 150 mg or 300 mg tablet
- Combivir®: Tablet, 300 mg ZDV + 150 mg 3TC

Advantages
- ZDV associated with decreased risk for HIV transmission
- ZDV used more often than other drugs for PEP for healthcare personnel (HCP)
- Serious toxicity rare when used for PEP
- Side effects predictable and manageable with antimotility and antiemetic agents
- Can be used by pregnant HCP
- Can be given as a single tablet (Combivir®) twice daily

Disadvantages
- Side effects (especially nausea and fatigue) common and might result in low adherence
- Source-patient virus resistance to this regimen possible
- Potential for delayed toxicity (oncogenic/teratogenic) unknown

● **Zidovudine (Retrovir®; ZDV; AZT) + emtricitabine (Emtriva™; FTC)**

Preferred dosing
- ZDV: 300 mg twice daily or 200 mg three times daily, with food; total: 600 mg daily in 2-3 divided doses
- FTC: 200 mg (one capsule) once daily

Dosage forms
- ZDV: 100 mg capsule, 300 mg tablet
- FTC: 200 mg capsule

FTC general comments
- Nucleoside analogue; same structure as 3TC, except fluoride residue at position 5 on pyrimidine ring
- Same resistance and safety profile as 3TC
- No apparent advantage over 3TC; tolerability and virologic response rates appear better than regimens containing ddl + *d4T*

Advantages
- ZDV: See above
- FTC
- Convenient (once daily)
- Well tolerated
- Long intracellular half-life (~40 hours)

Disadvantages
- ZDV: See above
- FTC
  - Rash perhaps more frequent than with 3TC
  - No long-term experience with this drug
  - Cross resistance to 3TC
  - Hyperpigmentation among non-Caucasians with long-term use: 3%

Tenofovir DF (Viread®; TDF) + lamivudine (Epivir®; 3TC)

Preferred dosing
- TDF: 300 mg once daily
- 3TC: 300 mg once daily or 150 mg twice daily

Dosage forms
- TDF: 300 mg tablet
- 3TC: 150 mg or 300 mg tablet

Advantages
- 3TC: See above
- TDF
  - Convenient dosing (single pill once daily)
  - Resistance profile activity against certain thymidine analogue mutations
  - Well tolerated

Disadvantages
- TDF
  - Same class warnings as nucleoside reverse transcriptase inhibitors (NRTIs)
  - Drug interactions
  - Increased TDF concentrations among persons taking atazanavir and lopinavir/ritonavir; need to monitor patients for TDF-associated toxicities
- Preferred dosage of atazanavir if used with TDF: 300 mg + ritonavir 100 mg once daily + TDF 300 mg once daily

Tenofovir DF (Viread®; TDF) + emtricitabine (Emtriva™; FTC); available as Truvada™

Preferred dosing
- TDF: 300 mg once daily
- FTC: 200 mg once daily
- Truvada™: One tablet daily

Dosage forms
- TDF: 300 mg tablet
- FTC: See FTC
- Truvada™ (TDF 300 mg plus FTC 200 mg)

Advantages
- FTC: See above
- TDF
  — Convenient dosing (single pill once daily)
  — Resistance profile activity against certain thymidine analogue mutations
  — Well tolerated

Disadvantages
- TDF
- Same class warnings as nucleoside reverse transcriptase inhibitors (NRTIs)
  — Drug interactions
  — Increased TDF concentrations among persons taking atazanavir and lopinavir/ritonavir; need to monitor patients for TDF-associated toxicities
- Preferred dosage of atazanavir if used with TDF: 300 mg + ritonavir 100 mg once daily + TDF 300 mg once daily

ALTERNATE BASIC REGIMENS

Lamivudine (Epivir®; 3TC) + stavudine (Zerit®; d4T)

Preferred dosing
- 3TC: 300 mg once daily or 150 mg twice daily
- d4T: 40 mg twice daily (can use lower doses of 20-30 mg twice daily if toxicity occurs; equally effective but less toxic among HIV-infected patients with peripheral neuropathy); 30 mg twice daily if body weight is <60 kg

Dosage forms
- 3TC: 150 mg or 300 mg tablet
- d4T: 15 mg, 20 mg, 30 mg, and 40 mg tablet

Advantages
- 3TC: See above
- d4T: Gastrointestinal (GI) side effects rare

Disadvantages
- Possibility that source-patient virus is resistant to this regimen
- Potential for delayed toxicity (oncogenic/teratogenic) unknown

Emtricitabine (Emtriva™; FTC) + stavudine (Zerit®; d4T)

Preferred dosing
- FTC: 200 mg daily
- d4T: 40 mg twice daily (can use lower doses of 20-30 mg twice daily if toxicity occurs; equally effective but less toxic among HIV-infected patients with peripheral neuropathy); 30 mg twice daily if body weight is <60 kg

Dosage forms
- FTC: See above
- d4T: See above

Advantages
- 3TC and FTC: See above; d4T's GI side effects rare

Disadvantages
- Potential that source-patient virus is resistant to this regimen
- Unknown potential for delayed toxicity (oncogenic/teratogenic) unknown

● **Lamivudine (Epivir®; 3TC) + didanosine (Videx®; ddI)**

Preferred dosing
- 3TC: 300 mg once daily or 150 mg twice daily
- ddI: Videx®; chewable/dispersible buffered tablets can be administered on an empty stomach as either 200 mg twice daily or 400 mg once daily. Patients must take at least two of the appropriate strength tablets at each dose to provide adequate buffering and prevent gastric acid degradation of ddI. Because of the need for adequate buffering, the 200 mg strength tablet should be used only as a component of a once-daily regimen. The dose is either 200 mg twice daily or 400 mg once daily for patients weighing >60 kg and 125 mg twice daily or 250 mg once daily for patients weighing >60 kg.

Dosage forms
- 3TC: 150 mg or 300 mg tablet
- ddI: 25 mg, 50 mg, 100 mg, 150 mg, or 200 mg buffered white tablets

Advantages
- 3TC: See above
- ddI: Once daily dosing option

Disadvantages
- Tolerability: Diarrhea more common with buffered preparation than with enteric-coated preparation
- Associated with toxicity: Peripheral neuropathy, pancreatitis, and lactic acidosis
- Must be taken on empty stomach except with TDF
- Drug interactions
- 3TC: See above

Emtricitabine (Emtriva™; FTC) + didanosine (Videx®; ddI)

Preferred dosing
- FTC: 200 mg once daily
- ddI: See above

Dosage forms
- FTC: See above
- ddI: See above

Advantages
- FTC: See above
- ddI: See above

Disadvantages
- Tolerability: Diarrhea more common with buffered preparation than with enteric-coated preparation
- Associated with toxicity: Peripheral neuropathy, pancreatitis, and lactic acidosis
- Must be taken on empty stomach except with TDF
- Drug interactions
- FTC: See above

PREFERRED EXPANDED REGIMEN

Basic regimen plus:

Lopinavir / Ritonavir (Kaletra™; LPV/RTV)

Preferred dosing
- LPV/RTV: 400 mg/100 mg = 3 capsules twice daily with food

Dosage forms
- LPV/RTV: 133 mg/33 mg capsules

Advantages
- Potent HIV protease inhibitor
- *Generally well tolerated*

Disadvantages
- Potential for serious or life-threatening drug interactions
- Might accelerate clearance of certain drugs, including oral contraceptives (requiring alternative or additional contraceptive measures for women taking these drugs)
- Can cause severe hyperlipidemia, especially hypertriglyceridemia
- GI (eg, diarrhea) events common

ALTERNATE EXPANDED REGIMEN

Basic regimen plus one of the following:

Atazanavir **(Reyataz®; ATV) ± ritonavir (Norvir®; RTV)**

Preferred dosing
- ATV: 400 mg once daily, unless used in combination with TDF, in which case ATV should be boosted with RTV, preferred dosing of ATV 300 mg + RTV: 100 mg once daily

Dosage forms
— ATV: 100 mg, 150 mg, and 200 mg capsules
— RTV: 100 mg capsule

Advantages
- Potent HIV protease inhibitor
- Convenient dosing – once daily
- Generally well tolerated

Disadvantages
- Hyperbilirubinemia and jaundice common
- Potential for serious or life-threatening drug interactions
- Avoid coadministration with proton pump inhibitors
- Separate antacids and buffered medications by 2 hours and H_2-receptor antagonists by 12 hours to avoid decreasing ATV levels
- Caution should be used with ATV and products known to induce PR prolongation (eg, diltiazem)

Fosamprenavir **(Lexiva™; FOSAPV) ± ritonavir (Norvir®; RTV)**

Preferred dosing
- FOSAPV: 1400 mg twice daily (without RTV)
- FOSAPV: 1400 mg once daily + RTV 200 mg once daily
- FOSAPV: 700 mg twice daily + RTV 100 mg twice daily

Dosage forms
- FOSAPV: 700 mg tablets
- RTV: 100 mg capsule

Advantages
- Once daily dosing when given with ritonavir

Disadvantages
- GI side effects common
- Multiple drug interactions. Oral contraceptives decrease fosamprenavir concentrations.
- Incidence of rash in healthy volunteers, especially when used with low doses of ritonavir. Differentiating between early drug-associated rash and acute seroconversion can be difficult and cause extraordinary concern for the exposed person.

Indinavir **(Crixivan®; IDV) ± ritonavir (Norvir®; RTV)**

Preferred dosing
- IDV 800 mg + RTV 100 mg twice daily without regard to food

Alternative dosing
- IDV 800 mg every 8 hours, on an empty stomach

Dosage forms
- IDV: 200 mg, 333 mg, and 400 mg capsule
- RTV: 100 mg capsule

Advantages
- Potent HIV inhibitor

Disadvantages
- Potential for serious or life-threatening drug interactions
- Serious toxicity (eg, nephrolithiasis) possible; consumption of 8 glasses of fluid/day required
- Hyperbilirubinemia common; must avoid this drug during late pregnancy
- Requires acid for absorption and cannot be taken simultaneously with ddl, chewable/dispersible buffered tablet formulation (doses must be separated by ≥1 hour)

Saquinavir (Invirase®; SQV) + ritonavir (Norvir®; RTV)

Preferred dosing
- SQV: 1000 mg (given as Invirase®) + RTV 100 mg, twice daily
- SQV: Five capsules twice daily + RTV: One capsule twice daily

Dosage forms
- SQV (Invirase®): 200 mg
- RTV: 100 mg capsule

Advantages
- Generally well-tolerated, although GI events common

Disadvantages
- Potential for serious or life-threatening drug interactions
- Substantial pill burden

Nelfinavir (Viracept®; NFV)

Preferred dosing
- NFV: 1250 mg (2 x 625 mg or 5 x 250 mg tablets), twice daily with a meal

Dosage forms
- NFV: 250 mg or 625 mg tablet

Advantages
- Generally well-tolerated

Disadvantages
- Diarrhea or other GI events common
- Potential for serious and/or life-threatening drug interactions

Efavirenz (Sustiva®; EFV)

Preferred dosing
- EFV: 600 mg daily, at bedtime

Dosage forms
- EFV: 50 mg, 100 mg, 200 mg capsules
- EFV: 600 mg tablet

Advantages
- Does not require phosphorylation before activation and might be active earlier than other antiretroviral agents (a theoretic advantage of no demonstrated clinical benefit)
- Once daily dosing

Disadvantages
- Drug associated with rash (early onset) that can be severe and might rarely progress to Stevens-Johnson syndrome
- Differentiating between early drug-associated rash and acute seroconversion can be difficult and cause extraordinary concern for the exposed person
- Central nervous system side effects (eg, dizziness, somnolence, insomnia, or abnormal dreaming) common; severe psychiatric symptoms possible (dosing before bedtime might minimize these side effects)
- Teratogen; should not be used during pregnancy
- Potential for serious or life-threatening drug interactions

ANTIRETROVIRAL AGENTS GENERALLY NOT RECOMMENDED FOR USE AS PEP

Nevirapine (Viramune®; NVP)

Disadvantages
- Associated with severe hepatotoxicity (including at least one case of liver failure requiring liver transplantation in an exposed person taking PEP)
- Associated with rash (early onset) that can be severe and progress to Stevens-Johnson syndrome
- Differentiating between early drug-associated rash and acute seroconversion can be difficult and cause extraordinary concern for the exposed person
- Drug interactions: Can lower effectiveness of certain antiretroviral agents and other commonly used medicines

Delavirdine (Rescriptor®; DLV)

Disadvantages
- Drug associated with rash (early onset) that can be severe and progress to Stevens-Johnson syndrome
- Multiple drug interactions

Abacavir (Ziagen®; ABC)

Disadvantages
- Severe hypersensitivity reactions can occur, usually within the first 6 weeks
- Differentiating between early drug-associated rash/hypersensitivity and acute seroconversion can be difficult

Zalcitabine (Hivid®; ddC)

Disadvantages
- Three times a day dosing
- Tolerability
- Weakest antiretroviral agent

ANTIRETROVIRAL AGENT FOR USE AS PEP ONLY WITH EXPERT CONSULTATION

Enfuvirtide (Fuzeon™; t20)

Preferred dosing
- T20: 90 mg (1 mL) twice daily by subcutaneous injection

Dosage forms
- T20: Single-dose vial, reconstituted to 90 mg/mL
- EFV: 600 mg tablet

Advantages
- New class
- Unique viral target; to block cell entry
- Prevalence of resistance low

Disadvantages
- Twice-daily injection
- Safety profile: Local injection site reactions
- Never studied among antiretroviral-naive or HIV-negative patients
- False-positive EIA HIV antibody tests might result from formation of anti-T20 antibodies that cross-react with anti-gp41 antibodies

HAZARDOUS COMMUNICATION

Communication regarding the dangers of bloodborne infections through the use of labels, signs, information, and education is required. Storage locations (eg, refrigerators and freezers, waste containers) that are used to store, dispose of, transport, or ship blood or other potentially infectious materials require labels. The label background must be red or bright orange with the biohazard design and the word biohazard in a contrasting color. The label must be part of the container or affixed to the container by permanent means.

Education provided by a qualified and knowledgeable instructor is mandated. The sessions for employees must include:
- accessible copies of the regulation
- general epidemiology of bloodborne diseases
- modes of bloodborne pathogen transmission
- an explanation of the exposure control plan and a means to obtain copies of the written plan
- an explanation of the tasks and activities that may involve exposure
- the use of exposure prevention methods and their limitations (eg, engineering controls, work practices, personal protective equipment)
- information on the types, proper use, location, removal, handling, decontamination, and disposal of personal protective equipment
- an explanation of the basis for selection of personal protective equipment

- information on the HBV vaccine, including information on its efficacy, safety, and method of administration and the benefits of being vaccinated (ie, the employee must understand that the vaccine and vaccination will be offered free of charge)
- information on the appropriate actions to take and persons to contact in an emergency involving exposure to blood or other potentially infectious materials
- an explanation of the procedure to follow if an exposure incident occurs, including the method of reporting the incident
- information on the postexposure evaluation and follow-up that the employer is required to provide for the employee following an exposure incident
- an explanation of the signs, labels, and color coding
- an interactive question-and-answer period

RECORD KEEPING

The OSHA Final Rule requires that the employer maintain both education and medical records. The medical records must be kept confidential and be maintained for the duration of employment plus 30 years. They must contain a copy of the employee's HBV vaccination status and postexposure incident information. Education records must be maintained for 3 years from the date the program was given.

OSHA has the authority to conduct inspections without notice. Penalties for cited violation may be assessed as follows.

Serious violations. In this situation, there is a substantial probability of death or serious physical harm, and the employer knew, or should have known, of the hazard. A violation of this type carries a mandatory penalty of up to $7000 for each violation.

Other-than-serious violations. The violation is unlikely to result in death or serious physical harm. This type of violation carries a discretionary penalty of up to $7000 for each violation.

Willful violations. These are violations committed knowingly or intentionally by the employer and have penalties of up to $70,000 per violation with a minimum of $5000 per violation. If an employee dies as a result of a willful violation, the responsible party, if convicted, may receive a personal fine of up to $250,000 and/or a 6-month jail term. A corporation may be fined $500,000.

Large fines frequently follow visits to laboratories, physicians' offices, and healthcare facilities by OSHA Compliance Safety and Health Offices (CSHOS). Regulations are vigorously enforced. A working knowledge of the final rule and implementation of appropriate policies and practices are imperative for all those involved in the collection and analysis of medical specimens.

Effectiveness of universal precautions in averting exposure to potentially infectious materials has been documented. 7 Compliance with appropriate rules, procedures, and policies, including reporting exposure incidents, is a matter of personal professionalism and prudent self-preservation.

Footnotes

1. Henderson DK, Fahey BJ, Willy M, et al, "Risk for Occupational Transmission of Human Immunodeficiency Virus Type 1 (HIV-1) Associated With Clinical Exposures. A Prospective Evaluation," *Ann Intern Med*, 1990, 113(10):740-6.

2. Niu MT and Margolis HS, "Moving Into a New Era of Government Regulation: Provisions for Hepatitis B Vaccine in the Workplace, *Clin Lab Manage Rev*, 1989, 3:336-40.

3. Bruning LM, "The Bloodborne Pathogens Final Rule — Understanding the Regulation," *AORN Journal,* 1993, 57(2):439-40.

4. "Rules and Regulations," *Federal Register,* 1994, 59(66):16360-3.

5. Schaffner W, Gardner P, and Gross PA, "Hepatitis B Immunization Strategies: Expanding the Target," *Ann Intern Med,* 1993, 118(4):308-9.

6. Fahey BJ, Beekmann SE, Schmitt JM, et al, "Managing Occupational Exposures to HIV-1 in the Healthcare Workplace," *Infect Control Hosp Epidemiol,* 1993, 14(7):405-12.

7. Wong ES, Stotka JL, Chinchilli VM, et al, "Are Universal Precautions Effective in Reducing the Number of Occupational Exposures Among Healthcare Workers?" *JAMA*, 1991, 265(9):1123-8.

THE FOLLOWING INFORMATION IS A SERIES OF QUICK NOTES REGARDING OCCUPATIONAL EXPOSURES, RISKS, AND FOLLOW-UP PROCEDURES

Hepatitis B Vaccination Recommended

For all potentially exposed employees
At no cost to employees
At a reasonable time and place
Administered by a licensed healthcare professional (HCP)
Within 10 days of initial assignment
Unless refused or not otherwise indicated
Waiver/declinations required, if refused
Full series and post immunization titer testing
MMWR ACIP recommendations for healthcare worker (HCW) Dec. 1999
3- to 6-day post-titer testing

Prevent Percutaneous Injuries

Use medical devices with safety features designed to prevent injuries and/or by using safer techniques:
- Self-sheathing needles
- Do not recap needles by hand
- Do not disengage needles from a reusable syringe
- Use disposable needle syringe systems
- Dispose of needles in appropriate sharps disposal containers

Avoid hand contact with sharps
Do not debride instruments on gauze by hand. Use a single-hand technique, such as:
- Cotton rolls taped to the instrument tray
- Use a commercial safe wipe device

Prevent Mucous Membrane and Skin Exposures

Avoid exposure to eyes, nose, mouth, or skin by using appropriate barriers:
- Gloves
- Eye and face protection
- Clinical attire

In Ohio, you must be vaccinated just before you can work – OSHA states within 10 days of employment.

OCCUPATIONAL EXPOSURE

Secondary Prevention
- Treat and contain the injury as soon as possible

If an Exposure Occurs
- Needlesticks and cuts/percutaneous injuries should be washed with soap and water
- Splashes to the nose, mouth, or skin should be flushed with water
- Eyes should be irrigated with clean water, saline, or sterile irrigants
- No scientific evidence shows that the use of antiseptics for wound care or squeezing the wound will reduce the risk of transmission of HIV; the use of a caustic agent such as bleach is not recommended

Postexposure Management (PEM) Steps

Step 1: Immediate wound decontamination and first aid; no extraordinary measure
Step 2: Report or communicate the incident to designated individual (maintain confidentiality); determine if the injury resulted in an exposure
Step 3: Discuss incident with source individual
Step 4: Initiate referral to the HCP
Step 5: Begin program of medical evaluation and follow-up (according to the most current recommendations of the USPHS)

Counseling

Source individual and exposed HCW
Informed consent
Confidentiality and disclosure
Risks of seroconversion:
- HIV: 0.3%
- HBV: 30% (6% to 35% estimates)
- HCV: 3% to 10%

Baseline Testing Injured Worker/Source Testing

Blood collection and baseline sero-status testing; establish sero-status at time of injury; this does not detect immediate infection from exposure

HIV, HBV, HCV testing

Blood can be drawn and stored for 90 days if the injured employee is not ready to have the blood tested at the time of the injury

See OSHA Employer Obligations: Postexposure Evaluations and Follow-up Requirements

Postexposure Medical Follow-up: Hepatitis B

Treat for HB_sAg

Treat exposed HCW

Vaccinated? — Current antibody status: Anti-Hb_sAg

Unvaccinated? — Hepatitis B immune globulin and dose #1 vaccines

Consider source HBV status

MMWR Morb Mortal Wkly Rep, 1991, 40(RR-13):1-25.

Postexposure Medical Follow-up: Hepatitis C

No pre- or postexposure recommendations

Baseline test for anti-HCV and ALT activity

Follow-up testing and liver function testing (4-6 months; HCV RNA at 4-6 weeks for early diagnosis)

No postexposure prophylaxis (PEP) with immune globulin or interferon

Treat chronic infection with interferon (USPHS)

MMWR Morb Mortal Wkly Rep, 1998, 47(RR-19):1-39.

Postexposure Medical Follow-up: HIV

Determine source status

Treat HCW/source

Follow-up according to source status and exposure

Follow current USPHS recommendations; *MMWR Morb Mortal Wkly Rep*, 1998, 47(RR-7):1-33.

What is the Risk of HIV Infection After Exposure?

Percutaneous: Average risk is 0.3% or about 1 in 300

Eye, nose, or mouth: Average risk is 0.1% or 1 in 1000

Skin: Average risk is 0.1%; higher if skin is damaged or contact is prolonged

Evaluate Risk of Percutaneous Exposure

Highest Risk: *BOTH* larger volume of blood (eg, deep injury, large-diameter needle previously in source patient's vein or artery) **AND** high titer of HIV (eg, source patient with acute retroviral illness or end-stage AIDS)

Increased Risk: *EITHER* larger volume of blood **OR** high titer of HIV

"In the absence of visible blood in the saliva, exposure to saliva from a person infected with HIV is not considered a risk for HIV transmission" – MMWR Morb Mortal Wkly Rep, 1998, 47(RR-7).

Follow-Up

– HIV antibody: Baseline, 6 weeks, 12 weeks, and 6 months postexposure

– Drug toxicity: Baseline and 2 weeks postexposure (CBC, renal, hepatic function)

Follow precautions to prevent transmission of HIV to others. Women should not breast-feed infants during the follow-up period.

Additional Information / Resources

CDC: 1-800-230-6039

– VOICE Information System: 888-232-3228

National Prevention Information Network

– Information Clearinghouse, HIV/AIDS and STDs: 1-800-458-5231

– HIV/AIDS Treatment Information Service: 1-800-448-0440

PEP Hotline: Toll-free: 888-448-4911

DENTAL MANAGEMENT CONSIDERATIONS FOR OSTEONECROSIS OF THE JAW (ONJ)

(Bisphosphonate-Related Osteonecrosis of the Jaw - BRONJ)

Diagnosis and Definition

- History of bisphosphonate therapy for bone disease of malignancy (usually breast, prostate, lung, or multiple myeloma) or for osteoporosis/osteopoenia or Paget's disease

- Intra oral pain is variable

- Complaint of roughness along the teeth or ridge (commonly seen along the mylohyoid ridge)

- History of dental procedures (extractions) (~60% post invasive procedure and ~40% spontaneous on mucosal areas away from teeth)

- Complaint of ill-fitting denture(s)

- Diagnosis made clinically with presence of exposed bone in the maxillofacial region for more than 8 weeks with no history of radiation therapy. Less than 8 weeks, the clinician must consider:
  - Spontaneous lingual mandibular sequestration with ulceration
  - Differential diagnosis
  - Trauma
  - Local malignancy
  - Periodontal disease

Suggested preventive dentistry before initiating chemotherapy, immunotherapy, or bisphosphonate therapy

- Remove abscessed and non-restorable teeth and teeth with severe periodontal disease involvement.

- Remove teeth with poor long-term prognosis.

- Functionally rehabilitate salvageable dentition, including endodontic therapy.

- Perform dental prophylaxis, caries control, and stabilizing restorative dental care.

- Examine dentures to ensure proper fit (dentures should be removed at night).

- Educate patients on oral self-care hygiene.

If a patient develops ONJ or BRONJ

- Consultations between oral surgeons/dental oncologists and the treating physician are strongly recommended.

- A nonsurgical approach is recommended to prevent further osseous injury (for example endodontics is preferred over extractions).

- Only minimal bony debridement to reduce sharp and rough surfaces to prevent further trauma to adjacent or opposing tissues is recommended.

- A removable appliance or protective stent may be used to protect exposed bone or adjacent tissues.

- Prophylactic antibiotic therapy may be considered for pain and disease control.

- We currently prescribe:

  – Amoxicillin 875 mg – Disp: 60 tabs – Sig: 1 tab bid

  – Chlorhexidine oral rinse – Disp: 1 bottle – Sig: 20 mL rinse and hold 30 sec bid

  In penicillin-allergic patients, clindamycin 300 mg tid can be substituted for amoxicillin; however, the patient must be cautioned to take with food due to GI risk with long-term clindamycin.

- Refill both prescriptions 2 times and re-evaluate in 3 months
  – Cultures should be taken for directed antimicrobial therapy.
  – Decisions regarding stopping BP therapy should be made in consultation between the treating oncologist and an oral and maxillofacial surgeon or dentist, taking into account the potential risk of further osteonecrosis versus the risk of skeletal complications.
  – Hyperbaric oxygen therapy is not recommended.
  – Biopsy is not recommended unless metastasis to the jaw is suspected.

ANIMAL AND HUMAN BITES GUIDELINES

The dentist is often confronted with early management of animal and human bites. The following protocols may assist in appropriate care and referral.

WOUND MANAGEMENT

- **Irrigation**: Critically important; irrigate all penetration wounds using 20 mL syringe, 19-gauge needle and >250 mL 1% povidone-iodine solution. This method will reduce wound infection by a factor of 20. When there is high risk of rabies, use veridical 1% benzalkonium chloride in addition to the 1% povidone-iodine. Irrigate would with normal saline after antiseptic irrigation.

- **Debridement:** Remove all crushed or devitalized tissue remaining after irrigation, minimize removal on face and over thin skin areas or anywhere you would create a worse situation than the bite itself already has; do not extend puncture wounds surgically – rather, manage them with irrigation and antibiotics.

- **Suturing**: Close most dog bites if <8 hours (<12 hours on face); do not routinely close puncture wounds, or deep or severe bites on the hands or feet, as these are at highest risk for infection. Cat and human bites should not be sutured unless cosmetically important. Wound edge freshening, where feasible, reduces infection, minimize sutures in the wound and used monofilament on the surface.

- **Immobilization**: Critical in all hand wounds; important for infected extremities.

- **Hospitalization/ I.V. Antibiotics**: Admit for I.V. antibiotics all significant human bites to the hand, especially closed fist injuries, and bites involving penetration of the bone or joint (a high index of suspicion is needed). Consider I.V. antibiotics for significant established wound infections with cellulitis or lymphangitis, any infected bite on the hand, any infected cat bite, and any infection in an immunocompromised or asplenic patient. Outpatient treatment with I.V. antibiotics may be possible in selected cases by consulting with infectious disease.

LABORATORY ASSESSMENT

- **Gram's Stain**: Not useful prior to onset of clinically apparent infection; examination of purulent material may show a predominant organism in established infection, aiding antibiotic selection; not warranted unless results will change your treatment.

- **Culture**: Not useful or cost-effective prior to onset of clinically apparent infection.

- **X-ray**: Whenever you suspect bony involvement, especially in craniofacial dog bites in very small children or severe bite/crush in an extremity; cat bites with their long needle-like teeth may cause osteomyelitis or a septic joint, especially in the hand or wrist.

IMMUNIZATIONS

- **Tetanus**: All bite wounds are contaminated. If not immunized in last 5 years or if not current in a child, give DPT, DT, Td, or TT as indicated. For absent or incomplete primary immunization, give 250 units tetanus immune globulin (TIG) in addition.

- **Rabies**: In the U.S. 30,000 persons are treated each year in an attempt to prevent 1-5 cases. Domestic animals should be quarantined for 10 days to prove need for prophylaxis. High-risk animal bites (85% of cases = bat, skunk, raccoon) usually receive treatment consisting of:

  — Human rabies immune globulin (HRIG): 20 units/kg I.M. (unless previously immunized with HDCV)

  — Human diploid cell vaccine (HDCV): 1 mL I.M. on days 0, 3, 7, 14, and 28 (unless previously immunized with HDCV – then give only first 2 doses)

BITE WOUNDS AND PROPHYLACTIC ANTIBIOTICS

- **Parenteral vs Oral**: If warranted, consider an initial I.V. dose to rapidly establish effective serum levels, especially if high risk, delayed treatment, or if patient reliability is poor.

- **Dog Bite**
  - Rarely get infected (~5%)
  - Infecting organisms: Staph coag negative, staph coag positive, alpha strep, diphtheroids, beta strep, *Pseudomonas aeruginosa*, gamma strep, *Pasteurella multocida*
  - Prophylactic antibiotics are seldom indicated. Consider for high risk wounds such as distal extremity puncture wounds, severe crush injury, bites occurring in cosmetically sensitive areas (eg, face), or in immunocompromised or asplenic patients.

- **Cat Bite**
  - Often get infected (~25% to 50%)
  - Infecting organisms: *Pasteurella multocida* (first 24 hours), coag positive staph, anaerobic cocci (after first 24 hours)
  - Prophylactic antibiotics are indicated in all cases.

- **Human Bite**
  - Intermediate infection rate (~15% to 20%)
  - Infecting organisms: Coag positive staph α, ß, γ strep, *Haemophilus*, *Eikenella corrodens*, anaerobic streptococci, *Fusobacterium*, *Veillonella*, bacteroides
  - Prophylactic antibiotics are indicated in almost all cases except superficial injuries.

BITE WOUND ANTIBIOTIC REGIMENS

	DOG BITE	**CAT BITE**	**HUMAN BITE**
Prophylaxis	No routine prophylaxis, consider if involves face or hand, or immunosuppressed or asplenic patients	Routine prophylaxis	Routine prophylaxis
Prophylactic antibiotic	Amoxicillin	Amoxicillin	Amoxicillin
Penicillin allergy	Doxycycline if >10 y or co-trimoxazole	Doxycycline if >10 y or co-trimoxazole	Doxycycline if >10 y or co-trimoxazole
OUTPATIENT ORAL ANTIBIOTIC TREATMENT (mild to moderate infection)			
Established infection	Amoxicillin and clavulanic acid	Amoxicillin and clavulanic acid	Amoxicillin and clavulanic acid
Penicillin allergy	Doxycycline if >10 y	Doxycycline if >10 y	Cephalexin[1] or clindamycin
OUTPATIENT PARENTERAL ANTIBIOTIC TREATMENT (moderate infection - single drug regimens)			
	Ceftriaxone	Ceftriaxone	Ceftriaxone
INPATIENT PARENTERAL ANTIBIOTIC TREATMENT			
Established infection	Ampicillin + cefazolin	Ampicillin + cefazolin	Ampicillin + clindamycin
Penicillin allergy	Cefazolin	Ceftriaxone	Cefotetan[1] or imipenem
Duration of Prophylactic and Treatment Regimens			
Prophylaxis: 5 days; Treatment: 10-14 days			

[1]Contraindicated if history of immediate hypersensitivity reaction (anaphylaxis) to penicillin

REFERENCES AND SELECTED READINGS

ANTIBIOTIC PROPHYLAXIS REFERENCES

"Advisory Statement. Antibiotic Prophylaxis for Dental Patients With Total Joint Replacement. American Dental Association; American Academy of Orthopaedic Surgeons," *J Am Dent Assoc,* 1997, 128(7):1004-8.

Baddour LM, Bettmann MA, Bolger AF, et al, "Nonvalvular Cardiovascular Device-Related Infections," *Circulation,* 2003, 108(16):2015-31.

Bashore TM, Cabell C, and Fowler V Jr, "Update on Infective Endocarditis," *Curr Probl Cardiol,* 2006, 31(4):274-352.

Bor DH and Himmelstein DU, "Endocarditis Prophylaxis for Patients With Mitral Valve Prolapse. A Quantitative Analysis," *Am J Med,* 1984, 76(4):711-7.

Brause BD, "Infections Associated With Prosthetic Joints," *Clin Rheum Dis,* 1986, 12(2):523-36.

Brennan MT, Kent ML, Fox PC, et al, "The Impact of Oral Disease and Nonsurgical Treatment on Bacteremia in Children," *J Am Dent Assoc,* 2007, 138(1):80-5.

Burton JP, Chilcott CN, Moore CJ, et al, "A Preliminary Study of the Effect of Probiotic Streptococcus salivarius K12 on Oral Malodour Parameters," *J Appl Microbiol,* 2006, 100(4):754-64.

Ching DW, Gould IM, Rennie JA, et al, "Prevention of Late Haematogenous Infection in Major Prosthetic Joints," *J Antimicrob Chemother,* 1989, 23(5):676-80.

Clemens JD and Ransohoff DF, "A Quantitative Assessment of Pre-Dental Antibiotic Prophylaxis for Patients With Mitral-Valve Prolapse," *J Chron Dis,* 1984, 37(7):531-44.

Dajani AS, Taubert KA, Wilson W, et al, "Prevention of Bacterial Endocarditis. Recommendations by the American Heart Association," *JAMA,* 1997, 277(22):1794-801.

Dajani AS, Bisno AI, Chung KJ, et al, "Prevention of Bacterial Endocarditis. Recommendations by the American Heart Association," *JAMA,* 1990, 264(22): 2919-22.

Dajani AS, Bawdon RE, and Berry MC, "Oral Amoxicillin as Prophylaxis for Endocarditis: What Is the Optimal Dose?" *Clin Infect Dis,* 1994, 18(2):157-60.

Durack DT, "Antibiotics for Prevention of Endocarditis During Dentistry: Time to Scale Back?" *Ann Intern Med,* 1998, 129(10):829-31.

Durack DT, "Prevention of Infective Endocarditis," *N Engl J Med,* 1995, 332(1):38-44.

Duval X, Alla F, Hoen B, et al, "Estimated Risk of Endocarditis in Adults With Predisposing Cardiac Conditions Undergoing Dental Procedures With or Without Antibiotic Prophylaxis," *Clin Infect Dis,* 2006, 42(12):e102-7.

Gould FK, Elliott TS, Foweraker J, et al, "Guidelines for the Prevention of Endocarditis: Report of the Working Party of the British Society for Antimicrobial Chemotherapy," *J Antimicrob Chemother,* 2006, 57(6):1035-42.

Hanssen AD, Osmon DR, and Nelson CL, "Prevention of Deep Prosthetic Joint Infection," *J Bone Joint Surg,* 1996, 78:458-71.

Johnson DP and Bannister GC, "The Outcome of Infected Arthroplasty of the Knee," *J Bone Joint Surg (Br),* 1986, 68(2):289-91.

Karchmer AW, "Infective Endocarditis," *Braunwald's Heart Disease: A Textbook Of Cardiovascular Medicine,* 7th ed, Zipes D, Libby P, and Bonow RO, eds, Philadelphia, PA: WB Saunders Co, 2005, 1633-58.

Krasse P, Carlsson B, Dahl C, et al, "Decreased Gum Bleeding and Reduced Gingivitis by the Probiotic Lactobacillus reuteri," *Swed Dent J,* 2006, 30(2):55-60.

Little J, "The American Heart Association's Guidelines for the Prevention of Bacterial Endocarditis: A Critical Review," *Gen Dent,* 1998, 46:508-15.

Little JW, Falace DA, Miller CS, et al, "Prosthetic Implants," *Dental Management of the Medically Compromised Patient,* 5th ed, Mosby, St Louis: MO, 1997, 602-17.

Lockhart PB, "The Risk for Endocarditis in Dental Practice," *Periodontol* 2000, 2000, 23:127-35.

Meurman JH and Stamatova I, "Probiotics: Contributions to Oral Health," *Oral Dis,* 2007, 13(5):443-5.

Moreillon P, Francioli P, Overholser D, et al, "Mechanisms of Successful Amoxicillin Prophylaxis of Experimental Endocarditis Due to Streptococcus Intermedius," *J Infect Dis,* 1986, 154(5):801-7.

Pallasch TJ, "A Critical Appraisal of Antibiotic Prophylaxis," *Int Dent J,* 1989, 39(3):183-96.

"Risks for and Prevention of Infective Endocarditis," *Cardiology Clinics - Diagnosis and Management of Infective Endocarditis,* Child JS, ed, Philadelphia, PA: WB Saunders Co, 1996, 14:327-43.

Skiest DJ and Coykendall AL, "Prosthetic Hip Infection Related to a Dental Procedure Despite Antibiotic Prophylaxis," *Oral Surg Oral Med Oral Pathol Oral Radiol Endod,* 1995, 79(5):661-3.

Strom BL, Abrutyn E, Berlin JA, et al, "Dental and Cardiac Risk Factors for Infective Endocarditis. A Population-Based, Case-Control Study," *Ann Intern Med,* 1998, 129(10):761-9.

Strom BL, Abrutyn E, Berlin JA, et al, "Prophylactic Antibiotics to Prevent Infective Endocarditis? Relative Risks Re-Assessed," *J Investig Med,* 1996, 44:229.

Teughels W, Van Essche M, Sliepen I, et al, "Probiotics and Oral Healthcare," *Periodontol* 2000, 2008, 48:111-47.

Twetman S and Stecksén-Blicks C, "Probiotics and Oral Health Effects in Children," *Int J Paediatr Dent,* 2008, 18(1):3-10.

Wahl M, "Myths of Dental-Induced Prosthetic Joint Infections," *Clin Infect Dis,* 1995, 20(5):1420-5.

Wilson W, Taubert KA, Gewitz M, et al, "Prevention of Infective Endocarditis: Guidelines From the American Heart Association: A Guideline From the American Heart Association Rheumatic Fever, Endocarditis, and Kawasaki Disease Committee, Council on Cardiovascular Disease in the Young, and the Council on Clinical Cardiology, Council on Cardiovascular Surgery and Anesthesia, and the Quality of Care and Outcomes Research Interdisciplinary Working Group," *Circulation,* 2007, 116(15):1736-54.

Wynn RL, "Amoxicillin Update," *Gen Dent,* 1991, 39(5):322, 324, 326.

Wynn RL and Bergman SA, "Antibiotics and Their Use in the Treatment of Orofacial Infections, Part I," *Gen Dent,* 1994, 42(5): 398, 400, 402.

Wynn RL, "New Erythromycins," *Gen Dent,* 1996, 44(4):304-7.

Wynn RL, Meiller TF, and Crossley HL, "New Guidelines for the Prevention of Bacterial Endocarditis. American Heart Association," *Gen Dent,* 1997, 45(5):426-8, 430-4.

AUTOMATED EXTERNAL DEFIBRILLATOR (AED)

"AAOHN Position Statement: Use of Automatic External Defibrillators, " *AAOHN J,* 1998, 46(7):324.

Alexander RF, "The Automated External Defibrillator: Single Citation Lifesaving Device for Medical Emergencies," *J Am Dent Assoc,* 1999, 130(6):837-45; *J Am Dent Assoc,* 1999, 130(8):1-162 [published erratum].

Bocka JJ, "Automatic External Defibrillators," *Ann Emerg Med,* 1997, 18(12):1264-8.

Cobb LA, Eliastam M, Kerber RE, et al, "Report of the American Heart Association Task Force on the Future of Cardiopulmonary Resuscitation," *Circulation,* 1992, 85(6):2346-55.

Cummins RO and Thies W, "Encouraging Early Defibrillation: The American Heart Association and Automated External Defibrillation," *Ann Emerg Med*, 1990, 19(11):1245-8.

Cummins RO, "Emergency Medical Services and Sudden Cardiac Arrest: The "Chain of Survival" Concept," *Ann Rev Public Health,* 1993, 14:313-33.

Cummins RO, White RD, and Pepe PE, "Ventricular Fibrillation, Automatic External Defibrillators, and the United States Food and Drug Administration: Confrontation Without Comprehension," *Ann Emerg Med,* 1995, 26(5):621-31.

Eisenberg MS, Pantridge JF, Cobb LA, "The Revolution and Evolution of Prehospital Cardiac Care," *Arch Intern Med,* 1996, 156(15):1611-9.

Fromm RE Jr and Varon J, "Automated External Versus Blind Manual Defibrillation by Untrained Lay Rescuers," *Resuscitation,* 1997, 33(3):219-21.

Gliner BE and White RD, "Electrocardiographic Evaluation of Defibrillation Shocks Delivered to Out-of-Hospital Sudden Cardiac Arrest Patients," *Resuscitation,* 1999, 41(2):133-44.

Kellermann AL, Hackman BB, Somes G, et al, "Impact of First-Responder Defibrillation in an Urban Emergency Medical Services System," *JAMA,* 1993, 270(14):1708-13.

Kerber RE, Becker LB, Bourland JD, et al, "Automatic External Defibrillators for Public Access Defibrillation: Recommendations for Specifying and Reporting Arrhythmia Analysis Algorithm Performance, Incorporating New Waveforms, and Enhancing Safety. A Statement for Health Professionals From the American Heart Association Task Force on Automatic External Defibrillation, Subcommittee on AED Safety and Efficacy," *Circulation,* 1997, 495(6):1677-82.

Link MS, Atkins DL, Passman RS, et al, "Electrical Therapies: Automated External Defibrillators, Defibrillation, Cardioversion, and Pacing," 2010 American Heart Association Guidelines for Cardiopulmonary Resuscitation and Emergency Cardiovascular Care, *Circulation,* 2010, 122:S706-S719, doi: 10.1161/CIRCULATIONAHA. 110.970954.

Malamed SF, *Medical Emergencies in the Dental Office,* 6th ed, Mosby, 2007.

Mancini ME and Kaye W, "AEDs. Changing the way you Respond to Cardiac Arrest. Automatic External Difibrillators," *Am J Nurs,* 1999, 99(5):26-30.

O'Hearn P, "Early Defibrillation: Lessons Learned," *J Cardiovasc Nurs,* 1996, 10(4):24-36.

Poole JE, White RD, Kantz KG, et al, "Low-Energy Impedance-Compensating Biphasic Waveforms Terminate Ventricular Fibrillation at High Rates in Victims of Out-of-Hospital Cardiac Arrest. LIFE Investigators," *J Cardiovasc Electrophysiol,* 1997, 8(12):1373-85.

Smith KL, Cameron PA, Peeters A, et al, "Automatic External Defibrillators: Changing the way we Manage Ventricular Fibrillation," *Med J Aust,* 2000, 172(8):384-8.

Varon J, Sternbach GL, Marik PE, et al, "Automatic External Defibrillators: Lessons From the Past, Present, and Future," *Resuscitation,* 1999, 41(3):219-23.

Weisfeldt ML, Kerber RE, McGoldrick RP, et al, "Public Access Defibrillation. A Statement for Healthcare Professionals From the American Heart Association Task Force on Automatic External Defibrillation," *Circulation,* 1995, 92(9):2763.

DENTAL OFFICE MEDICAL EMERGENCIES: ORAL MEDICINE BOOKS, CHAPTERS & MANUSCRIPTS

Alexander RE, "A Prevention-Oriented Approach to Dental Office Emergencies," *US Navy Med,* 1979, 70(10):16-20.

Alexander RE, "The Automated External Cardiac Defibrillator: Lifesaving Device for Medical Emergencies," *J Am Dent Assoc,* 1999, 130(6):837-45.

Anderson PE, "Effectively Handling Medical Emergencies," *Dent Econ,* 1989, 79(11):54, 56, 58-60.

Anderson K, "Preparing for Medical Complications in the Dental Office," *CDS Rev,* 1996, 89(3):28-30.

Assael LA, "Acute Cardiac Care in Dental Practice," *Dent Clin North Am,* 1995, 39(3):555-65.

Bavitz JB, "Emergency Management of Hypoglycemia and Hyperglycemia," *Dent Clin North Am,* 1995, 39(3):587-94.

Becker DE, "Management of Immediate Allergic Reactions," *Dent Clin North Am,* 1995, 39(3):577-86.

Bennett JD, "Emergency Drug Therapy. Drugs and Routes of Administration," *Dent Clin North Am,* 1995, 39(3):501-21.

Bradley BE, Dworin AM, and Gobetti JP, "Medical Emergencies in Dental Practice. Part II: Emergency Kit and Equipment," *J Mich Dent Assoc,* 1979, 61(3):199-203.

Briceno de Martinez B, "The Medical Emergency in the Dental Office," *Acta Odontol Venez,* 1987, 25(2):365-9.

Capuano A and Bertini L, "Cardiovascular Emergencies in Dental Surgery," *G Anest Stomatol,* 1990, 19(4):11-7.

Debien BA, Lienhart P, Le Dantec, et al, "Indispensable Resuscitation Equipment," *Rev Odontostomatol (Paris),* 1991, 20(5):439-46.

Dietz ER, "Dental Office Emergencies," *Dent Assist,* 1978, 47(6):30-5, 40.

Dworin AM and Gobetti JP, "Medical Emergencies in Dental Practice. Part III-Cardiovascular Emergencies," *J Mich Dent Assoc,* 1979, 61(4):255-60.

Fast TB, Martin MD, and Ellis TM, "Emergency Preparedness: A Survey of Dental Practitioners," *J Am Dent Assoc,* 1986, 112(4):499-501.

Freeman NS, King RA, Plezia RA, et al, "Office Emergencies: An Outline of Causes, Symptoms, and Treatment," *J Am Dent Assoc,* 1977, 94(1):91-6.

Gitelman JM, "Medical Emergencies in the Dental Office," *J Dist Columbia Dent,* 1977, Soc:13-5.

Goodman RA and Solomon SL, "Transmission of Infectious Diseases in Outpatient Health Care Settings," *JAMA,* 1991, 265(18):2377-81.

Goupil MT, "Occupational Health and Safety Emergencies," *Dent Clin North Am,* 1995, 39(3):637-47.

Harnisch H, "Medical Treatment of Emergencies in the Dental Office," *Zahnarztl Prax,* 1987, 38(12):451-3.

Imbert M and Fuilla C, "Cardiopulmonary Arrest," *Rev Odontostomatol (Paris),* 1991, 20(5):373-6.

Jimenez Vazquez P and Garcia Luna M, "Recommendations for Basic Emergency Equipment in the Dental Office," *Pract Odontol,* 1991, 12(7):35-9.

King DR, "Dental Office Emergencies-Update on the Basics," *Dent Surv,* 1978, 54(10):50-3.

Legens M and Roche Y, "Behavioral Disturbances and Psychosomatic Manifestations," *Rev Odontostomatol (Paris),* 1991, 20(5):401-4.

Linke H, "Medical Emergencies in the Dental Office," *Dtsch Stomatol,* 1970, 20(10):776-87.

Lipp M, Kubota Y, Malamed SF, et al, "Management of an Emergency: To Be Prepared for the Unwanted Event," *Anesth Pain Control Dent,* 1992, 1(2):90-102.

Malamed SF, "Back to Basics: Emergency Medicine in Dentistry," *J Calif Dent Assoc,* 1997, 25(4):285-6, 288-94.

Malamed SF, "Managing Medical Emergencies," *J Am Dent Assoc,* 1993, 124(8):40-53.

Malamed SF, *Medical Emergencies in the Dental Office,* 6th ed, Mosby, 2007.

McCarthy FM, "A Minimum Medical Emergency Kit," *Compendium,* 1994, 15(2):214, 216, 218-20 passim; quiz 224.

Norris LH, "Early Recognition Limits in In-Office Emergencies," *J Mass Dent Soc,* 1994, 43(3):19-23.

Norris LH, "Prepare for Medical Emergencies," *J Mass Dent Soc,* 1994, 43(2):27-9.

Parlato M and Del Duca P, "Emergency Situations in the Dental Office. Prevention and Organization," *Arch Stomatol (Napoli),* 1990, 31(4):767-73.

Parsons JR, "The Principles of Diagnosis," *Dent Clin North Am,* 1974, 18(1):3-23.

Pelissier A, "Translaryngeal Trocar, Alternative to Tracheotomy in the Dental Office," *Rev Odontostomatol (Paris),* 1991, 20(5):431-7.

Phero JC, "Maintaining Preparedness for the Life-Threatening Office Medical Emergency," *Dent Econ,* 1991, 81(5):47-8, 50.

Piecuch JF and Lieblich SE, "Neurologic Emergencies," *Dent Clin North Am,* 1995, 39(3):567-75.

Roberts MW and Morrill GS, "Medical Emergencies and a Standardized Emergency Kit for the Dental Office," *J Acad Gen Dent,* 1972, 20(5):36-9.

Robson TJ and Robb N, "Emergency Drugs in Dental Practice: A Minimalistic View," *SAAD Dig,* 1996, 13(1):3-11.

Rosenberg MB and Phero JC, "Resuscitation of the Pediatric Patient," *Dent Clin North Am,* 1995, 39(3):663-76.

Saef SH, "Assessment of the Medical Emergency," *Dent Clin North Am,* 1995, 39(3):487-99.

Schijatschky M, "Incidents in the Dental Office Which Could Endanger the Life of the Patient," *Quintessenza,* 1970, 1(2):5-12

Straka E, Pickles T, Bartley M, et al, "Office Environment Hazards Committee report. Recommended Standards for: Control of Environmental Hazards; Establishment and Maintenance of Records; Management of Medical Emergencies," *J Oreg Dent Assoc,* 1983, 52(4):31-4.

Thompson I, "Emergency Treatment in Australia," *Anesth Pain Control Dent,* 1992, 1(3):167-70.

Waitley NG, "Your Patient at Risk-Office Emergencies," *J Mo Dent Assoc,* 1976, 56(4):39-44.

Wakeen LM, "Dental Office Emergencies: Do You Know Your Legal Obligations?" *J Am Dent Assoc,* 1993, 124(8):54-8.

Woodworth JV, "Recognition and Treatment of Medical Emergencies in the Dental Office," *J Am Dent Assoc,* 1970, 81(4):887-93.

Young ER, "The Dental Office Medical Emergency: What Do I Do?" *J Can Dent Assoc,* 1994, 60(2):117-20.

EMERGENCY MEDICINE: TEXTS AND REFERENCES

Adler JN, Plantz SH, Stearns DA, et al, *Emergency Medicine,* 1st ed, Baltimore, MD: Lippincott Williams & Wilkens, 1999.

American Heart Association, Heartsaver Plus, Emergency Cardiovascular Care Programs, 1997.

Bates B, Bickley LS, and Hoekelman RA, *Physical Examination and History Taking,* 6th ed, Philadelphia, PA: J. B. Lippincott Company, 1995.

Bosker G, Weins D, and Sequeira M, *The 60-Second EMT: Rapid BLS/ALs Assessment, Diagnosis & Triage,* 2nd ed, St. Louis, MO: Mosby-Year Book Inc, 1996

Bricker SL, Langlais RP, and Miller CS, *Oral Diagnosis, Oral Medicine, and Treatment Planning,* Philadelphia, PA: Lea & Febiger, 1994.

Burrell KH, Byrne BE, Ganzberg S, et al, *ADA Guide to Dental Therapeutics,* 1st ed, Chicago, IL: ADA Publishing Co, Inc, 1998.

Campbell J E (ed), *Basic Trauma Life Support for Paramedics and Advanced Ems Providers,* 3rd ed, Prentice-Hall, 1998.

"Protection Against Viral Hepatitis: Recommendations of the Immunization Practices Advisory Committee," *MMWR, Morb Mortal Wkly Rep,* 1990, 39(RR-2).

"Public Health Service Inter-Agency Guidelines for Screening Donors of Blood, Plasma, Organs, Tissues, and Semen for Evidence of Hepatitis B and Hepatitis C," *MMWR Morb Mortal Wkly Rep,* 1991, 40(RR-4).

"Hepatitis B Virus: A Comprehensive Strategy for Eliminating Transmission in the United States Through Universal Childhood Vaccination: Recommendations of the Advisory Committee on Immunization Practices," *MMWR Morb Mortal Wkly Rep,* 1991, 40(RR-13).

"Recommended Infection-Control Practices for Dentistry," *MMWR Morb Mortal Wkly Rep,* 1993, 42(RR-8).

"Prevention of Hepatitis A Through Active or Passive Immunization - Recommendations of the Advisory Committee on Immunization Practices," *MMWR Morb Mortal Wkly Rep,* 1996, 45(RR-15):1-30.

Cummins RO and Graves J, *ACLS Scenarios: Core Concepts for Case-Based Learning,* 2nd ed, Mosby-Year Book, 1995.

Einzig M (ed), *The Baby & Child Emergency First Aid Handbook: Simple Step-By-Step Instructions for the Most Common Childhood Emergencies,* Meadowbrook Press, 1992.

Eversole LR, *Oral Medicine: A Pocket Guide,* Philadelphia: W. B. Saunders Company, 1996 .

Jenkins JL, Loscalzo J, and Braen GR, *Manual of Emergency Medicine,* 3rd ed, Boston: Little, Brown and Company, 1995.

Little JW, Falace DA, Miller CS, et al, *Dental Management of the Medically Compromised Patient,* 5th ed, St. Louis: Mosby-Year Book, Inc., 1997.

Lynch MA, Brightman VJ, and Greenberg MS (ed), *Burket's Oral Medicine: Diagnosis and Treatment,* 9th ed, Philadelphia: J. B. Lippincott Company, 1994.

Malamed SF, *Medical Emergencies in the Dental Office,* 6th ed, Mosby, 2007.

"Management of Hepatitis C," *NIH Consensus Statement,* 1997, 15(3).

O'Keefe MF, Limmer D, Grant HD, et al, *Brady Emergency Care,* 8th ed, Brady Games, 1998.

Polk DA, Hunt RC, Gardner M, et al, *Advanced Life Support Skills,* Mosby-Year Book, 1993.

Skinner D, Swain A, Peyton R, et al, *Cambridge Textbook of Accident and Emergency Medicine,* Cambridge University Press, 1997.

Sonis ST, Fazio RC, and Fang L, *Principles and Practice of Oral Medicine,* 2nd ed, Philadelphia: W. B. Saunders Company, 1995.

Sprigings D, Chambers J, Jeffrey A, et al, *Acute Medicine: A Practical Guide to the Management of Medical Emergencies,* 2nd ed, Blackwell Science Inc, 1995.

Stillwell SB, *Quick Critical Care Reference,* 3rd ed, St. Louis: Mosby-Year Book Inc., 1998.

Taylor RV, Key CB, Trach M, et al, *Advanced Cardiac Care in the Streets,* Lippincott Williams & Wilkins Publishers, 1998.

Terezhalmy GT and Batizy LG (ed), *Urgent Care in the Dental Office: An Essential Handbook,* Quintessence Publishing Co, 1998.

Tintinalli JE, Ruiz E, and Krome RL (ed), *Emergency Medicine: A Comprehensive Study Guide,* 4th ed, McGraw Hill Text, 1995.

White RD, Paturas JL, McSwain Jr NE, et al, *The Basic EMT: Comprehensive Prehospital Patient Care,* Mosby-Year Book, 1996.

Winchester J and Winchester LP, *Clinical Management of Poisoning and Drug Overdose,* 3rd ed, W. B. Saunders Co, 1998.

Zydio S, *The American Medical Association Handbook of First Aid & Emergency Care,* Random House, 1990.

OCCUPATIONAL EXPOSURE TO BLOODBORNE PATHOGENS REFERENCES

Buehler JW and Ward JW, "A New Definition for AIDS Surveillance," *Ann Intern Med,* 1993, 118(5):390-2.

Brown JW and Blackwell H, "Complying With the New OSHA Regs, Part 1: Teaching Your Staff About Biosafety," *MLO,* 1992, 24(4)24-8. Part 2: "Safety Protocols No Lab Can Ignore," 1992, 24(5):27-9. Part 3: "Compiling Employee Safety Records That Will Satisfy OSHA," 1992, 24(6):45-8.

Department of Labor, Occupational Safety and Health Administration, "Occupational Exposure to Bloodborne Pathogens; Final Rule (29 CFR Part 1910.1030), " *Federal Register,* December 6, 1991, 64004-182.

Gold JW, "HIV-1 Infection: Diagnosis and Management," *Med Clin North Am,* 1992, 76(1):1-18.

"Hepatitis B Virus: A Comprehensive Strategy for Eliminating Transmission in the United States Through Universal Childhood Vaccination," Recommendations of the Immunization Practices Advisory Committee (ACIP), *MMWR Morb Mortal Wkly Rep,* 1991, 40(RR-13):1-25.

"Mortality Attributable to HIV Infection/AIDS — United States", *MMWR Morb Mortal Wkly Rep,* 1991, 40(3):41-4.

National Committee for Clinical Laboratory Standards, "Protection of Laboratory Workers From Infectious Disease Transmitted by Blood, Body Fluids, and Tissue," NCCLS Document M29-T, Villanova, PA: NCCLS, 1989, 9(1).

"Nosocomial Transmission of Hepatitis B Virus Associated With a Spring-Loaded Fingerstick Device — California," *MMWR Morb Mortal Wkly Rep,* 1990, 39(35):610-3.

Polish LB, Shapiro CN, Bauer F, et al, "Nosocomial Transmission of Hepatitis B Virus Associated With the Use of a Spring-Loaded Fingerstick Device," *N Engl J Med,* 1992, 326(11):721-5.

"Recommendations for Preventing Transmission of Human Immunodeficiency Virus and Hepatitis B Virus to Patients During Exposure-Prone Invasive Procedures," *MMWR Morb Mortal Wkly Rep,* 1991, 40(RR-8):1-9.

"Update: Acquired Immunodeficiency Syndrome — United States," *MMWR Morb Mortal Wkly Rep,* 1992, 41(26):463-8.

"Update: Transmission of HIV Infection During an Invasive Dental Procedure — Florida," *MMWR Morb Mortal Wkly Rep,* 1991, 40(2):21-7, 33.

"Update: Universal Precautions for Prevention of Transmission of Human Immunodeficiency Virus, Hepatitis B Virus, and Other Bloodborne Pathogens in Healthcare Settings," *MMWR Morb Mortal Wkly Rep,* 1988, 37(24):377-82, 387-8.

OSTEONECROSIS OF THE JAW REFERENCES

Advisory Task Force on Bisphosphonate-Related Osteonecrosis of the Jaws, American Association of Oral and Maxillofacial Surgeons, "American Association of Oral and Maxillofacial Surgeons Position Paper on Bisphosphonate-Related Osteonecrosis of the Jaws," *J Oral Maxillofac Surg,* 2007, 65(3):369-76.

ADA Council on Scientific Affairs. Expert Panel Recommendations: Dental Management of Patients on Oral Bisphosphonate Therapy, June 2006. Available at: http://www.ada.org/prof/resources/pubs/jada/reports/report_bisphosphonate.pdf.

American Dental Association Council on Scientific Affairs, "Dental Management of Patients Receiving Oral Bisphosphonate Therapy: Expert Panel Recommendations," *J Am Dent Assoc,* 2006, 137(8):1144-50.

Arthritis and Allied Conditions: A Textbook of Rheumatology, Vol 1, 15th ed, Koopman WJ and Moreland LW, eds, Philadelphia, PA: Lippincott, Williams and Wilkins, 2005, 1448.

Badros A, Weikel D, Salama A, et al, "Osteonecrosis of the Jaw in Multiple Myeloma Patients: Clinical Features and Risk Factors," *J Clin Oncol,* 2006, 24(6):945-52.

Black DM, Delmas PD, Eastell R, et al, "Once-Yearly Zoledronic Acid for Treatment of Postmenopausal Osteoporosis," *N Engl J Med,* 2007, 356(18):1809-22.

Bone HG, Hosking D, Devogelaer JP, et al, "Ten Years' Experience With Alendronate for Osteoporosis in Postmenopausal Women," *N Engl J Med,* 2004, 350(12):1189-99.

Durie BG, Katz M, and Crowley J, "Osteonecrosis of the Jaw and Bisphosphonates," *N Engl J Med,* 2005, 353(1):99-102.

Grant BT, Amenedo C, Freeman K, et al, "Outcomes of Placing Dental Implants in Patients Taking Oral Bisphosphonates: A Review of 115 Cases," *J Oral Maxillofac Surg,* 2008, 66(2):223-30.

Hoff AO, Toth BB, Altundag K, et al, "Osteonecrosis of the Jaw in Patients Receiving Intravenous Bisphosphonate Therapy," *J Clin Oncol,* 2006, 24:8528; available at http://meeting.jco.org/content/abstract/24/18_suppl/8528.

Jeffcoat MK, "Safety of Oral Bisphosphonates: Controlled Studies on Alveolar Bone," *Int J Oral Maxillofac Implants,* 2006, 21(3):349-53.

Johnston CC Jr, Bjarnason NH, Cohen FJ, et al, "Long-Term Effects of Raloxifene on Bone Mineral Density, Bone Turnover, and Serum Lipid Levels in Early Postmenopausal Women: Three-Year Data From 2 Double-Blind, Randomized, Placebo-Controlled Trials," *Arch Intern Med,* 2000, 160(22):3444-50.

Marx RE, Cillo JE Jr, and Ulloa JJ, "Oral Bisphosphonate-Induced Osteonecrosis: Risk Factors, Prediction of Risk Using Serum CTX Testing, Prevention, and Treatment," *J Oral Maxillofac Surg,* 2007, 65(12):2397-410.

Marx RE, *Oral and Intravenous Bisphosphonate-Induced Osteonecrosis of the Jaws: History, Etiology, Prevention and Treatment,* Chicago, IL: Quintessence Publishing Company, 2007, 87-91.

Marx RE, Sawatari Y, Fortin M, et al, "Bisphosphonate-Induced Exposed Bone (Osteonecrosis/Osteopetrosis) of the Jaws: Risk Factors, Recognition, Prevention, and Treatment," *J Oral Maxillofac Surg,* 2005, 63(11):1567-75.

Mavrokokki T, Cheng A, Stein B, et al, "Nature and Frequency of Bisphosphonate-Associated Osteonecrosis of the Jaws in Australia," *J Oral Maxillofac Surg,* 2007, 65(3):415-23.

Migliorati CA, Casiglia J, Epstein J, et al, "Managing the Care of Patients With Bisphosphonate-Associated Osteonecrosis: An American Academy of Oral Medicine Position Paper," *J Am Dent Assoc,* 2005, 136(12):1658-68.

Ott SM, "Long-Term Safety of Bisphosphonates," J Clin Endocrinol Metab, 2005, 90(3):1294-301.

Reginster J, Minne HW, Sorensen OH, et al, "Randomized Trial of the Effects of Risedronate on Vertebral Fractures in Women With Established Postmenopausal Osteoporosis. Vertebral Efficacy With Risedronate Therapy (VERT) Study Group," *Osteoporos Int,* 2000, 11(1):83-91.

Rosen HN, Moses AC, Garber J, et al, "Serum CTX: A New Marker of Bone Resorption That Shows Treatment Effect More Often Than Other Markers Because of Low Coefficient of Variability and Large Changes With Bisphosphonate Therapy," *Calcif Tissue Int,* 2000, 66(2):100-3.

Ruggiero SL and Drew SJ, "Osteonecrosis of the Jaws and Bisphosphonate Therapy," *J Dent Res,* 2007, 86(11):1013-21.

Ruggiero SL, Fantasia J, and Carlson E, "Bisphosphonate-Related Osteonecrosis of the Jaw: Background and Guidelines for Diagnosis, Staging and Management," *Oral Surg Oral Med Oral Pathol Oral Radiol Endod,* 2006, 102(4):433-41.

Ruggiero SL, Mehrotra B, Rosenberg TJ, et al, "Osteonecrosis of the Jaws Associated With the Use of Bisphosphonates: A Review of 63 Cases," *J Oral Maxillofac Surg,* 2004, 62(5):527-34.

Ruggiero S, Gralow J, Marx RE, et al, "Practical Guidelines for the Prevention, Diagnosis, and Treatment of Osteonecrosis of the Jaw in Patients With Cancer," *Journal of Oncology Practice,* 2006, 2(1):7-14.

Scheper MA, Badros A, Chaisuparat R, Cullen KJ, Meiller TF. Role of Zoledronic Acid in the Apoptotic Cell Death of Oral Fibroblasts and Epithelial Cells: A Mechanism of Bisphosphonate-Associated Osteonecrosis. *British Journal of Haematology,* 2009, Mar,144(5):667-76. Epub 2008 Nov 20.PMID: 19036117

Scheper MA, Badros A, Salama AR, et al, "A Novel Bioassay Model to Determine Clinically-Significant Bisphosphonate Levels," *Support Care Cancer,* 2009, Aug 4. [Epub ahead of print] PMID: 19653010

Scully C, Madrid C, and Bagan J, "Dental Endosseous Implants in Patients on Bisphosphonate Therapy," *Implant Dent,* 2006, 15(3):212-8.

Starck WJ and Epker BN, "Failure of Osseointegrated Dental Implants After Diphosphonate Therapy for Osteoporosis: A Case Report," *Int J Oral Maxillofac Implants,* 1995, 10(1):74-8.

Tarassoff P and Hei YJ, "Osteonecrosis of the Jaw and Bisphosphonates," *N Engl J Med,* 2005, 353:101-2.

Verispan, VONA, "The Top 200 Brand-Name Drugs by Units in 2006," *Drug Topics,* 2007.

Wang HL, Weber D, and McCauley LK, "Effect of Long-Term Oral Bisphosphonates on Implant Wound Healing: Literature Review and a Case Report," *J Periodontol,* 2007, 78(3):584-94.

Drug Information Handbook for Dentistry

The #1 Dental Reference with over 440,000 Copies Sold!

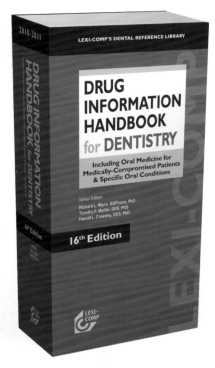

OVERVIEW:

The *Drug Information Handbook for Dentistry* is designed for all dental professionals seeking clinically-relevant information on medications, OTCs, and herbal products. Written by dentists for dentists, this best-selling resource includes dental-specific content on thousands of drugs, natural products, and dietary supplements.

THE BENEFITS:

Within this user-friendly resource, medications are alphabetically indexed by brand and generic names and index terms. Each drug monograph includes up to 38 unique fields of information, with dental-specific fields highlighted in red, a timesaving feature in an information-rich resource. Special sections dedicated to the medically-compromised patient, specific oral conditions, and sample prescriptions are included.

Lexi-Comp's *Drug Information Handbook for Dentistry* is excellent for chair-side use, supporting safe pharmacotherapy and improved patient care.

Updates to this Edition:

- 41 New Drug Monographs

- New Route-Specific Monographs: Systemic, Nasal, Ophthalmic, Otic, Topical

- Updated Oral Medicine Topics:
  - Rheumatoid Arthritis, Osteoarthritis, and Osteoporosis
  - Cardiovascular Diseases
  - Management of Patients Undergoing Cancer Therapy
  - Systemic Viral Diseases
  - Oral Pain
  - Ulcerative, Erosive, and Painful Oral Mucosal Disorders

- New Special Topic Sections:
  - Antiplatelet and Anticoagulation Considerations in Dentistry
  - Clinical Risk Related to Drugs Prolonging QT Interval
  - Osteonecrosis of the Jaw

- Updates to Appendix Information

Grow Your Referral Business
with a Lasting Reminder of Your Services

Give the gift of a Lexi-Comp dental reference manual *customized with your practice details.*

- ▶ **Promote your dental practice** and attract more patients

- ▶ **Increase visibility of your name** – daily use by dentists

- ▶ **Non-perishable gift** – used throughout the year

- ▶ **#1 dental references** – help dentists improve medication safety

- ▶ **Show appreciation** for your referring dentists

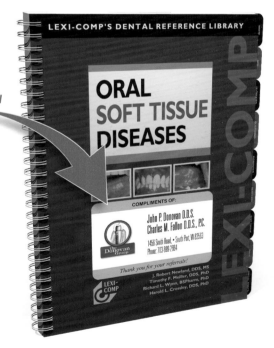

Building your patient base and growing referral business for your dental practice can be a challenge. With Lexi-Comp bookplates, marketing your practice couldn't be easier.

Customized with your contact details, Lexi-Comp bookplates let you show appreciation for your referring dentists while helping you grow business and increase revenue for your practice.

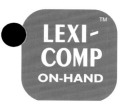

Lexi-Comp ON-HAND for Dentistry

Lexi-Comp ON-HAND for Dentistry provides instant access to point-of-care information on smartphones and handheld devices. *Updates to our content are available on a daily basis, ensuring you always have the most timely clinical information at your fingertips.*

Featuring Dental Lexi-Drugs, covering 8000 drugs and herbal products, with monographs containing up to 37 fields of information, including:

- U.S. Brand Names and Generic Names
- Special Alerts
- Use
- Local Anesthetic/Vasoconstrictor Precautions
- Effects on Dental Treatment

- Dental Dosing for Selected Drug Classifications
- Adverse Effects, Contraindications, Warnings/Precautions
- Drug Interactions
- Dental Comment

Lexi-Comp ON-HAND for PDA & Mobile Devices

  palm webOS Windows Mobile BlackBerry

On-the-go access to Lexi-Comp's dental-specific drug information!

Available for smartphones and other mobile devices, Lexi-Comp's dental applications feature the full color images, charts, and appendices from our trusted dental print manuals!

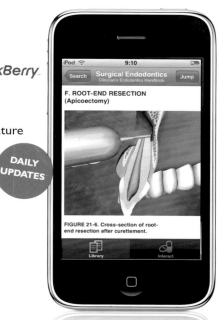

Available applications include:

Dental Lexi-Drugs *plus* Lexi-Interact
Price: $115 / 1 year subscription

Lexi-DENTAL SELECT
Price: $215 / 1 year subscription

Includes:
- Dental Lexi-Drugs
- Lexi-Interact
- Lexi-Drug ID
- Lexi-CALC
- Oral Soft Tissue Diseases
- Oral Hard Tissue Diseases
- Illustrated Handbook of Clinical Dentistry
- Dental Office Medical Emergencies
- The Little Dental Drug Booklet

Lexi-DENTAL COMPLETE
Price: $285 / 1 year subscription

Includes:
- Dental Lexi-Drugs
- Lexi-Interact
- Pediatric Lexi-Drugs
- Lexi-Drug ID
- Lexi-CALC
- Oral Soft Tissue Diseases
- Oral Hard Tissue Diseases
- Illustrated Handbook of Clinical Dentistry
- Dental Office Medical Emergencies
- The Little Dental Drug Booklet
- Clinician's Endodontic Handbook
- Manual of Clinical Periodontics
- Manual of Dental Implants
- Oral Surgery for the General Dentist
- Advanced Protocols for Medical Emergencies
- Harrison's Practice
- Stedman's Medical Dictionary for the Health Professions and Nursing

For more information or to purchase visit:
www.lexi.com

ON-HAND
product tours:
www.lexi.com/individuals/tours

For more information, or to order any of these products, visit our web site or call Customer Service
www.lexi.com/dentistry
1-866-397-3433

See why more dentists are choosing Lexi-Comp.

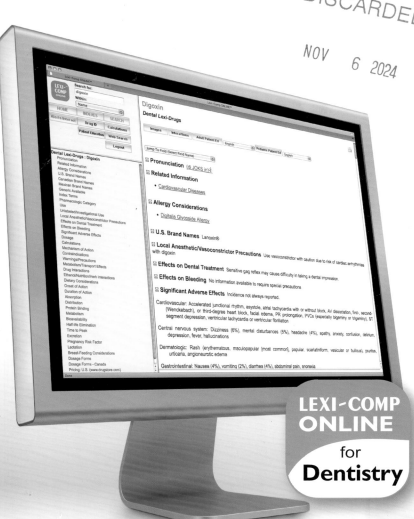

LEXI-COMP ONLINE for Dentistry

Lexi-Comp® ONLINE™ for Dentistry

provides dental professionals with dental-specific pharmacology information and drug interaction analysis tools to help ensure medication safety. This resource also features a complete dental reference library of information addressing dental conditions, clinical procedures including oral surgery videos, management of dental emergencies, and information regarding diagnosis, planning, and therapy for dental disciplines.

- **Searchable content** from the #1 rated *Drug Information Handbook for Dentistry* plus Lexi-Comp's entire dental reference library

- **Daily content updates** to ensure you stay current with the latest medication information

- A **dental-specific drug interaction screening tool** – designed to save time when checking for interactions and reduce the risk of adverse drug events

- **Trust Lexi-Comp** to recommend the safest medication when administering local anesthetics, antibiotics, and analgesics

Content Areas

- Drug Information
- Drug Interactions
- Dosing Calculations
- Natural Therapeutics
- Patient Education
- Dental Implants
- Oral Surgery
- Endodontics
- Periodontics
- Clinical Dentistry
- Oral Soft Tissue Diseases
- Oral Hard Tissue Diseases
- Medical Emergencies
- Office Finance

For more information, or to order any of these products, visit our web site or call Customer Service
www.lexi.com/dentistry
1-866-397-3433